THE Kama Sutra KITCHEN

AN APHRODISIAC RECIPE BOOK

ASHLEY APPLE

Photography by Vivek, Rob Perica and Nikki Ritcher
Editing by Adam Caplan and Ellen Gordon
Layout by Dean Fetzer, www.gunboss.com
Styling support by Eduardo Bettencourt
Cover design by Gary McCluskey

www.ashleyapple.com

DEDICATION

May everyone know immeasurable pleasure and experience a juicy sex life.

ACKNOWLEDGMENTS

I would like to thank all the people who made this book possible. The first giant step of editing was possible because of Adam Caplan. Thank you for smoothing out the edges. Thank you to my incredible models, Stephanie, Vidya, Satchita, Sophie, Eliza, Justine, Jason and Eduardo, for volunteering your bodies in the hot Thailand sun in the name of erotic art. Thank you Shelley for your enthusiasm and support. Thank you Courtney for being my number one cheerleader. Thank you to my parents, Ed and Sue, for believing in me and always being there. Thank you Vidya, for always shining eagerness my way. Thank you Andrew for inspiring my heart. Thank you Jenny for providing direction. Thank you Eduardo for encouraging me to be my most authentic Self. Thank you to all my incredible friends and family who have believed in me from the first vision. And lastly, thank you to all the people who indulged in my aphrodisiac creations over the years, for sampling, loving and sharing all the juicy feedback!

CONTENTS

For many centuries there has been a huge repressive energy around the topic of sex, sexuality and lovemaking. At the same time, the topic of sex and sexuality has a lot of dynamic energy and "movement" behind it.

The media uses sex to sell everything from movies to cars to household cleaning supplies! Even those people that renounce sex are still fiery and heated about the subject.

Whether you are open for explorative sexual adventures or conservatively discreet and virginal till marriage, the fact of the matter is that sex intrigues and inspires powerful energy.

If you are already titillated and intrigued, then hurry up and turn the page!

INTRODUCTION

This is a recipe book for creating aphrodisiac treats that increase sexual desire, passion, sensation, vitality, stamina and intensify orgasm. The secret to successful aphrodisiacs is in the alchemy of creating. In this book I introduce the concept of alchemy as a process of understanding the ingredients, the flavors, the textures of the raw ingredients while entertaining a sensual mood and loving state of consciousness. Everything about this book is designed to increase sensuality to support the proper mood while concocting aphrodisiac recipes. Allow the pictures to inspire your sensual urges. Most important, allow your hands to feel every ingredient with reverence and sensuality as they mix together to create edible bliss.

Each section of the book is short and sweet, designed to introduce you to the basic concepts of alchemy and herbal medicine. Reading about the individual herbs and super foods will give you a background for creating a specific effect. A lot of the recipes include raw cacao, or raw chocolate. I offer my own discoveries of blending and creating raw chocolate treats as a tool for simple kitchen alchemy. At the end of the book I have included suggestions for romantic bedroom menus. A guide to sexy seduction with your own home made aphrodisiacs!

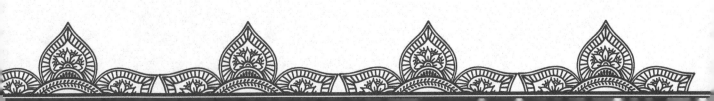

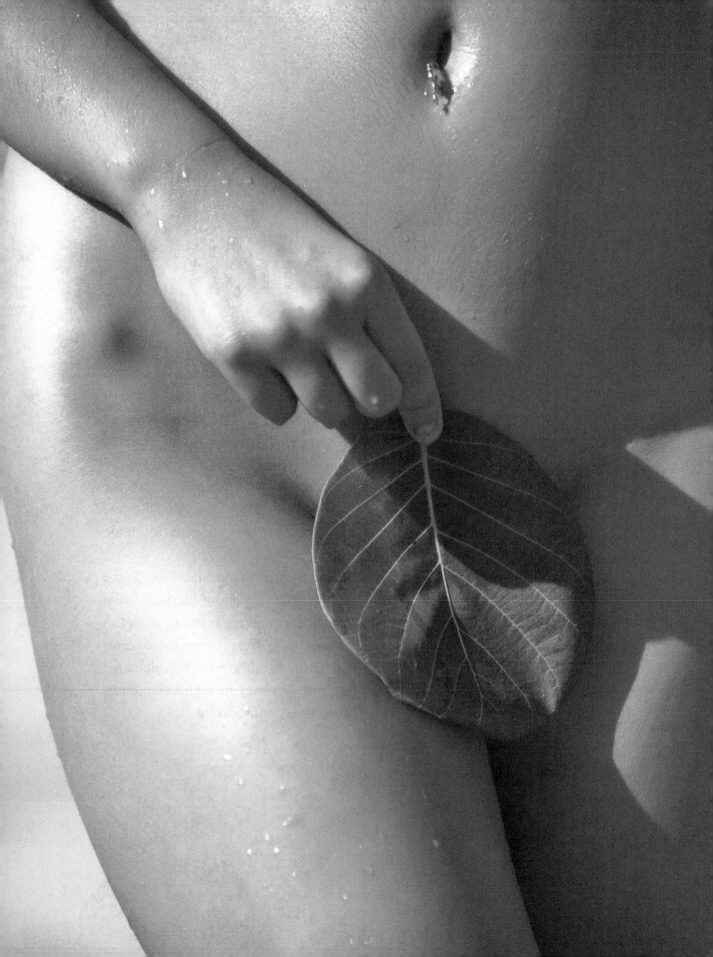

CHAPTER 1

APHRODISIAC QUEEN

When people find out what I do and learn about my passion for aphrodisiac plants they often ask me how I got started. I suppose it seems like a strange area to specialize in, although to me it came about quite naturally.

The story unfolds in the beginning of my herbal studies. I was always fascinated with the plant remedies that tasted good. As a child I used to hate all the foul tasting medicines that were a part of sickness and healing. With plant medicine I found there were many ways to make preparations taste good. Some were definitely more tasty and appealing than others. Sometimes with the right blending I could take an unpleasant tasting plant medicine and make it extremely tasty. Take herbal tea as an example. Drinking a daily tonic tea full of vitamins and minerals can taste like the lawn clippings from the front yard, but with the right mint, flowers, spices or fruit the same drink becomes a delicious beverage.

While I was attending herb school in Boulder, Colorado, I discovered a passion for creating herbal remedies that people actually desired and enjoyed! And then I met the plant damiana. It was love at first taste. The taste was floral and bitter with a sweet smelling aroma that intrigued me. damiana was the first plant I worked with on a daily basis. I tried it in tea, I made a tincture, sprinkled

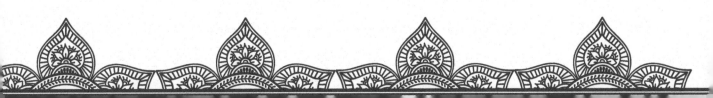

it inside an apple pie, and hey, I even put it in a pipe and smoked it! During my damiana infatuation I discovered beautiful Goddess-shaped glass bottles from Mexico filled with damiana liquor. The effects were amazing! I became infatuated with the idea that a plant can make me feel so good. I began to research other plants that had an immediate effect on the body's nervous system. I noticed myself consistently drawn more and more to the plants that affected sensuality. Perhaps it is due to my own Venetian, sensual nature that I found it so attractive or maybe it was just fate, but I quickly discovered an infatuation for plants that incited passion.

These days you can find all kinds of aphrodisiac/libido pills and formulas on line or in your local vitamin shop. Some of them really work, but I wonder: "How sexy is a pill?" I kept thinking about the essence of sexuality and decided that by making an aphrodisiac deliciously sensuous it would transform the person taking it and support a greater awakening of passion. What if eating a delicious mouth watering chocolate mousse in a sensual way could do as much or more as popping a pill?

What I have learned over the last ten years is the magic of alchemy and intention. When herbs are used for their medicinal effects and combined with delicious ingredients you have a pleasurable way of ingesting a medicinal preparation. By taking the plants and blending them into a desirable treat, it is possible to infuse the "medicine" with all kinds of potency. When you enjoy eating a "medicine" you increase its power and effects.

Over the years I took every opportunity to experiment on my friends. I brought some form of aphrodisiac to every potluck or social gathering. I would sit back and watch people enjoy them and notice how they ate them. Some recipes inspired people to eat slowly and savor the flavor. Sometimes the effects were fast and people would leave a gathering early, snuggled up against their lovers with that knowing look in their eyes thinking, "I can't wait to get you home!" I even hosted sensual theme parties in attempts to saturate my friends with love potions and plant passion. In time I became known for my passion inducing treats, and was often introduced as the "Tantric Aphrodisiac Love Goddess" or the "Aphrodisiac Queen."

Over the years I have finessed my recipes through trial and error. Some of the treats in this book have been inspiring sexual bliss for over ten years! I invite you to use these recipes to indulge your deepest passions and desires. May these recipes inspire you to discover new places and open to more love!

CHAPTER 2

AN APHRO-WHAT?

Aphrodisiac aph·ro·dis·i·ac (ăf'rə-dĭz'ē-āk', -dē'zē-)
adj.
Arousing, increasing, or intensifying sexual desire.*n.*
An aphrodisiac drug or food.

Aphrodisiac: A substance that increases, restores, arouses, enhances and intensifies sexual desire, urge, activity and potency. Aphrodisiacs are often used to stimulate erotic intentions and feelings.

What is an Aphrodisiac? An aphrodisiac is defined as any form of stimulation that arouses sexual excitement. Sexual desire and sensuality can be triggered by events, emotions, foods, herbs and spices. The word aphrodisiac comes from the name of the Greek Goddess Aphrodite. She is the Goddess of desire, love and beauty. Aphrodite had a son, Eros, also known as Cupid, the God of love, whose magical arrows could incite passionate love and tender affections. It is this idea that inspires many people to seek out help from plants and foods as a way of fanning the flames of ardor.

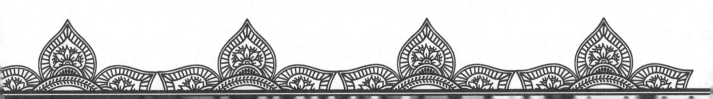

The search for aphrodisiacs is often fueled by the hope that our favorite exercise, sex, can be enhanced. It seems this desire for better sex is not limited by time, place, race or culture. Every major culture has searched out potential "love potions" that could increase desire and sexual drive. There are many plants that have a history among traditional people as potent aphrodisiacs and sexual tonics which tone the reproductive and hormonal systems. These "folk remedies" although unproven clinically have been used successfully for hundreds of years. A lot of the recipes in this book have been inspired by time tested plant combinations that were passed down through tradition and culture. Others are from my own formulating and experimentation.

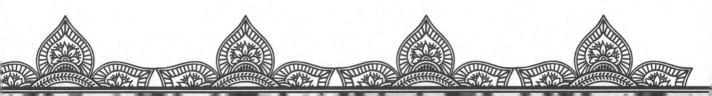

CHAPTER 3

TYPES OF APHRODISIACS

Aphrodisiacs can be classified into two main categories: the sensory oriented-those which affect through sight, sound, taste, touch and smell – and the internal which are consumed, such as: food, beverages, herbs, drugs, medicinal preparations and spices. This book focuses mainly upon the internal application of foods, herbs and spices for increasing sexual arousal.

We can divide the category of internal aphrodisiac plants into their sub-categories based on the different ways they act on the body. Some affect the physical body directly while others have more of an energetic effect. An example of a physical affect is the increase of circulation, the blood flow to the genitals. Another is when an aphrodisiac acts on the nervous system, relaxing the body and increasing sensitivity. Some plants balance the body and regulate the levels of various circulating hormones. For example, did you know that stress and tension create all kinds of chemicals in the body that may trigger certain hormones that keep you from being able to relax and express sexual energy?

These influential plants do not simply act on the physical body alone, but act upon the energy and emotional bodies as well. Many aphrodisiacs have a strong stimulating or psychedelic effect, making them a popular choice for those who wish to increase sensitivity and awareness of the subtle energies. To understand the different types of aphrodisiacs we first need to understand the different ways they can affect us and our energy.

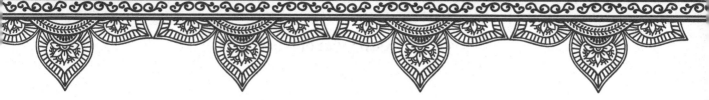

CHAPTER 4

SEXUALITY EXPRESSED BY THE PHYSICAL BODY

When we begin to analyze sexuality in the hopes of understanding what plants to use for increasing it, we find two different approaches: The physical and energetic.

Looking into the physical approach, we find there are many chemical reactions occurring in the body at any time. Some of the chemical reactions are responsible for the way we feel, the way we digest our food, the way our bodies build and breakdown cells and replenish energy. When we fall in love, achieve a great success or have an amazing orgasm the happy high we experience is often a result of several body chemicals getting released into the nervous system.

Science has identified many chemicals that affect how we feel. Tryptophan, serotonin, dopamine and phenylethylalamine are some of the popular ones you may have heard of. When we have large amounts of these chemicals circulating in the body we feel good, relaxed and even blissful. One of my favorite chemicals is anandamide. In Sanskrit the term "ananda" means bliss, so anandamide is the "bliss" chemical of the body. When we first meet someone and the attraction is

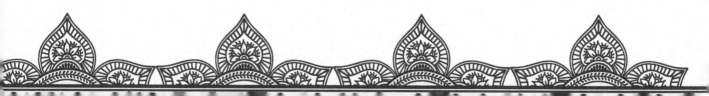

mutual we find ourselves on a natural high – life seems better, the sun is brighter and everything is just great. It also means we have anandamide circulating around our bloodstream.

Having a strong sexual appetite isn't just about the "happy" chemicals floating around inside the body. There are many chemicals in the body that can keep sexual interest or desire at a minimal level. For example, take the hormone cortisol, known as the stress hormone. If you were visiting the zoo when the lions escaped, and you saw one barreling down the sidewalk straight towards you, your nervous system would kick into gear. Your body would enter "fight or flight" mode, a reaction designed to keep you safe in life threatening situations. Bodily functions such as digestion and mind blowing orgasms are not priorities for survival in such stressful moments, so the body releases cortisol and other chemicals to shut them down and apply the energy where it is needed. Super human strength, speed and surprisingly quick thinking suddenly become available as you attempt to escape a grizzly death. So cortisol is great right! We need it to survive stressful situations. The problems come when there is too much cortisol in the bloodstream. It is not every day that a lion runs at us, but we constantly put ourselves in "flight or fight" mode, with all sorts of modern day stressors such as commuting, high-stress jobs and money obsession. Rarely do we give the body a chance to rebalance. Since we are always under stress, over a period of time we start to notice certain side effects such as chronic tension and chronically elevated stress hormone levels. Having cortisol levels constantly elevated will diminish anyone's sexual appetite. Lack of sexual desire and energy to perform are some of the most noticeable side effects of continual stress. Some aphrodisiacs work directly on reducing cortisol levels and providing support to a frayed nervous system.

There are many types of physical actions aphrodisiacs can have on the body; reducing stress hormones is just one. Another is nourishing the adrenal glands. A lot of traditional tonic aphrodisiacs help to normalize body functions, provide adrenal support and help bring the body into a state of balance. These tonics are called adaptogens because they are known for their rebalancing properties. I like to think of them as plants that help you "adapt" to life. Some aphrodisiacs increase circulation in the body. When by increasing blood flow to a certain area in the body you bring it fresh oxygen, nutrients and hormones that can help the body recharge and energize. Some aphrodisiac plants provide essential vitamins, minerals, amino acids and nutrients that are otherwise deficient in the average modern diet. In some cases low sex drive can be a simple side effect of poor nutrition.

Some aphrodisiacs provide a gentle irritation or sensation in the genitals. This is often referred to as "an itch I just need to scratch!" The itch is rather metaphorical here; it is not so much of an itchy feeling as a desire to want to touch and be touched.

My favorite aphrodisiacs have a physical effect on the nervous system. Some provide a sense of deep relaxation while others bring stimulation and charge. When the body is feeling deeply relaxed it is more sensitive to touch we are better able to feel energy. For times when you want the opposite effect, having the right tea can make you want to throw your lover onto the floor and wrestle, growl and play with such charge and intensity that you feel like a super hero. Whatever mood you are seeking to create, there are plants that can facilitate that desire.

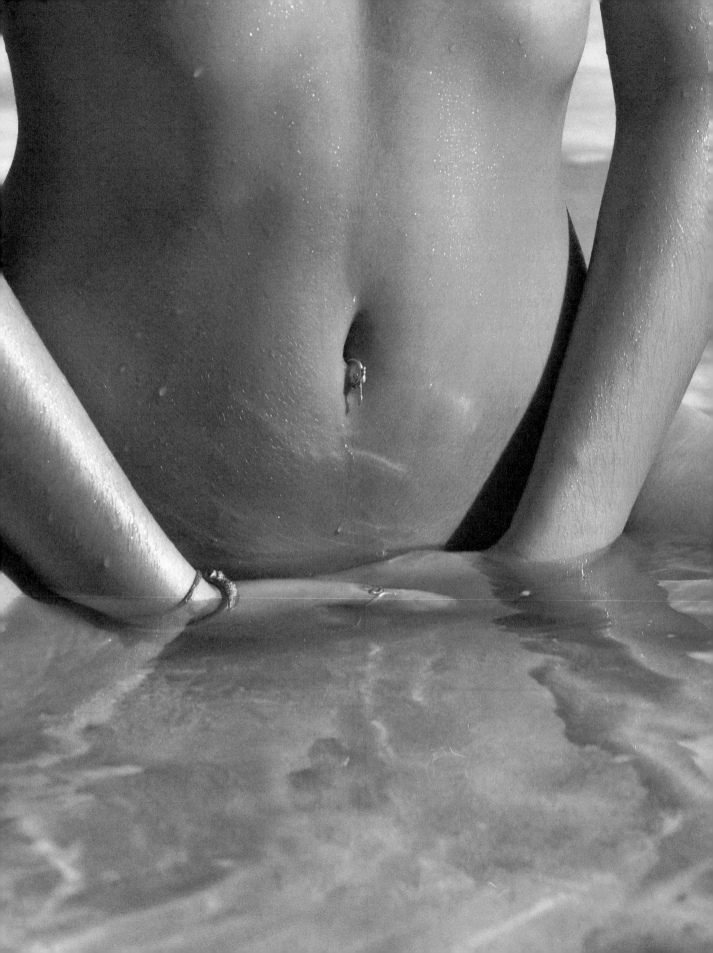

CHAPTER 5

THE ENERGY OF SEXUALITY

Let's look at the energetic aspect of sexuality. This concept tends to be harder to grasp because of our scientific minds and the way we are trained to experience the world. We are capable of extreme energetic sensitivity, but like a muscle that isn't put to use, our energetic sensors can be weak and small. If we want to become strong and develop the body we must exercise regularly and over time our body will change and so will our physical abilities.

The same is true of energy and our ability to perceive it. There are many tools for developing energetic sensitivity. Some of the most popular ones are meditation, martial arts and yoga. Some people are born with a natural sensitivity to energy, while others might spend months dedicated to a daily practice before they begin to experience their inner energetic world.

At some point everyone has experienced some form of energy. Have you ever been doing something when the hairs on the back of your neck suddenly rise up and you feel uncomfortable? Have you ever been thinking about someone and then the phone rings and you have a sensation, a knowing that it is that person? Ever noticed when we hug somebody sometimes that it just feels good, like we

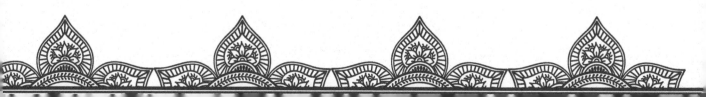

don't want to let go. All three examples are experiences in which our sensation of energy was affecting us.

Sometimes all we need is someone to share our stories with to find out that we have had all kinds of energetic experiences; we just didn't identify them as such. Having a close friend or a circle of support is essential for growing deeper in our awareness. I have often encouraged women to form small groups and gather to discuss and giggle over tea. Group gatherings are important for men, too, though men tend to bond over adrenaline-raising activities such as paint ball and sporting events.

Feeling your sexual energy can be a lot easier if you relax and open your mind. Let go of any preconceived notions of how things should be and witness everything you feel as if you were a child, new to the world. Some aphrodisiacs are especially good at increasing energetic sensitivity. If you want to increase your level of feeling, I recommend using aphrodisiacs that enhance energetic sensitivity with an open-minded partner. Having someone to share with and compare sensations with is valuable when you are learning to feel more within. I also recommend experimenting with practices from the Taoist or Tantric traditions to go deeper in your sexual exploration. Sexual Tantra is the study and practice of sublimating energy for the purpose of spiritual awakening. Mastering control over our sexual energy allows us to redirect it and utilize it for attaining presence, pure consciousness and love.

In Tantra the use of sexual energy is a powerful tool for stimulating the Kundalini Shakti. Kundalini Shakti is the dormant unconscious energy within every human being. The kundalini energy is often pictured as a sleeping snake, coiled at the base of the spine. As the energy is awakened it rises slowly up the spine passing through seven energy vortexes. These vortexes or wheels of energy are known as chakras. As the kundalini passes through each chakra, energy builds and changes. In yoga there are many breath control exercises and physical postures, designed to stimulate the awakening of the Kundalini. Aphrodisiacs can help facilitate this awakening along with a dedicated yoga practice and a desire to become more sensitive.

I have found incredible practices and resources in the study of Tantra yoga for controlling sexual energy. One of the main goals in Tantra is the conservation of all forms of energy, especially sexual energy. In Tantra, sexual energy is a gift with a powerful potential for generating energy that can be transmuted into higher states of consciousness. As energy moves from the lower chakras up along the spine you can experience high states of being.

I am often asked what sexual energy feels like as it moves up the spine. One way of relating to the sensation is remembering a time when you had to pee so badly you thought you would burst. Maybe you were on a long car ride and there was nowhere to stop. When you finally made it to the bathroom was there a momentary hesitation when your body didn't do anything, a buildup of sensation as you sat there, dying to pee and just waiting? Then, with a full body shiver and perhaps a stifled moan, you started to urinate, and for a brief moment a shiver ran up your spine. Slowly the sensation died down and you felt a deep sense of relaxation. It's not quite the same as a sexual response, but similar enough to give you something to base your experience on. That shiver and moan of painful pleasure was the release of built up energy from the lower body as it moved up the spine. The deep relaxation was an aftereffect of the movement of energy.

Aphrodisiacs can heighten your sexual experience by increasing the flow of energy in the body. An increase in energy between two people is often felt as chemistry. Chemistry, passion and desire are manifested forms of sexual energy, expressing itself through you as you connect. I often joked about my "poor medicated lovers" as never having a chance since I was always dosing them before we made it to the bedroom. Guiltless, I pass the knowledge on to you, for I guarantee nobody will ever complain about the mind-blowing orgasms they had with you all night. Trust me.

CHAPTER 6

THE GLORIOUS WORLD OF (TASTY) APHRODISIACS!

There are hundreds of plants, foods and spices traditionally used throughout history as aphrodisiacs. Some of the plants I have uncovered in my quest for the ultimate love potion have presented powerful effects yet their taste and flavor is less desirable when concocting edible bliss. For that reason alone I decided to include only the tasty aphrodisiacs in this book that should be a part of your Kama Sutra Kitchen. These plants are essential in your sexual alchemy!

I included two categories for each plant to help in a deeper, well-rounded understanding of the medicinal actions. The taste of the plant is helpful in understanding how to mix herbs together to create a culinary delight. For example if an herb is bitter adding it to honey or sweet nuts will help smooth out the flavor. The energy of a plant describes the effect it has on the body; warming, cooling, etc. A cold, frigid person would respond well to a hot spicy tea or warming chocolate treat. The more we understand the nature of each plant the easier it becomes to mix up an individualized aphrodisiac treat for our lover.

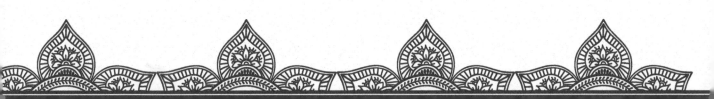

Damiana (Turnera aphrodisiaca)
Taste: floral, bitter and aromatic
Energy: warming

In Mexico, damiana has a long history of use among women. They would drink damiana tea several hours before making love to increase their desire. Chemically, this plant has been found to contain several alkaloids that directly stimulate the sex organs and libido. damiana acts powerfully upon the nervous system by being both stimulating and relaxing.

It stimulates the senses, awakening energetic sensitivity and sensation, while relaxing the body and allowing for greater opening and energy flow along the spine. Some women have claimed that it increases the sharpness of a female orgasm. A mild euphoric feeling and sensitivity to pleasure is often experienced by either ingesting and/or smoking the herb. This feeling can improve our sexual courage and help us release our inhibitions.

Maca (Lepidium meyenii)
Taste: slightly bitter, sweet, hint of vanilla malt
Energy: warming, building

Maca is often called Peruvian ginseng for its remarkable abilities to nourish and stimulate the body. Maca is a rich source of protein, vitamins and minerals. It is considered a food as well as a medicinal herb which has been traditionally used by those wanting to increase sexuality and increase overall energy. Maca's benefits include; supporting the proper functioning of the endocrine system and most of the body's glands that control sexual function, digestion, brain and the nervous system.

It has long been researched for its ability to increase sexual stamina and fertility (including an increased production of testosterone). Maca has a pleasant malt flavor that mixes easily into food or smoothies.

Maca can be taken on a daily basis to increase energy/stamina and balance hormones. (1tsp daily recommended dose) A slightly larger dose of Maca powder can be ingested in food or drink before sexual intimacy to increase a feeling of bliss, well-being, pleasure and joy. (1-2 tbs).

*A note of caution to men that experience premature ejaculation. Maca can increase the sensitivity of the penis by increasing histamines in the penile tissue. For those men struggling with premature ejaculation this herb can make you even more sensitive so experiment with awareness!

Guarana (Paullinia cupana)
Taste: smoky, slightly bitter, blends great with chocolate
Energetic: stimulating

The South American Indian tribes, especially the Guarani's, from whence the name is derived, dry and roast the seeds and mix them into a paste with water. This paste is then used in much the same way as chocolate to prepare various foods, drinks and medicines.

Guarana is used and well known for its stimulant action. It is reputed to increase mental alertness, to fight fatigue and also to increase stamina and physical endurance. Naturally high in caffeine, guarana can provide increased energy during long lovemaking sessions.

Guarana is reported to have 2.5 times more caffeine than coffee! The powdered seeds can also have large amounts of guaranine, a slight hallucinogenic, which can contribute a sacred feel to connecting with your partner. Take heed, a little goes a long way if you're looking for extra energy!

Kola Nut (Cola nitida)
Taste: bitter
Energetic: stimulating and energizing

Kola nut became popular when it was used as a main ingredient in the production of soft drinks, hence coca-cola! Its history as an aphrodisiac and energy stimulant is well documented by the West Africans. It has effects on the central nervous system similar to guarana, cacao and yerba mate, but with an even stronger euphoric effect.

It is a great herb to add to your formulas that require a little energy boost. If you are sensitive to caffeine or have high blood pressure this is one to be careful with!

Muira Puma (Ptychopetslum olscoides)
Taste: bitter
Energetic: drying, warming

Muira puma, also called "potency wood," in Brazil, has a long history in herbal medicine as an aphrodisiac and as a tonic for the nervous system. The root of muira puma is rich in fatty acids, essential oils and plant sterols. It has been used successfully as a neuromuscular tonic, and to treat PMS, menstrual symptoms and sexual impotency.

Traditionally, people would simmer the root bark in alcohol to extract all of the aphrodisiac properties. It can be prepared as a tea or consumed as powder, but I have received the most positive feedback from men who consumed a cordial with the heated Muira Puma alcohol extract. Look for the "Vira Elixir" recipe to find my tasty version!

Suma (Pfaffia paniculata)
Taste: sweet and slightly bitter
Energetic: neutral

In South America, suma is known as **Para Toda**, which means "for all things." Like maca and ginseng, suma is widely used as an adaptogen. Suma is an important herbal remedy in the folk medicine of several indigenous Indian tribes today. It has been used as a tonic and an aphrodisiac for over 300 years.

It is considered a tonic for the cardiovascular system, the central nervous system, the reproductive system, and the digestive system, and, it is used to treat hormonal disorders, sexual dysfunction and sterility. In European herbal medicine Suma is used to treat infertility, menopausal and menstrual symptoms and to minimize the side effect of birth control medications.

Suma has a light vanilla flavor making it another excellent herb to use in foods. I find it to be a wonderful addition to tonic recipes since it seems to be most effective over a period of time.

Catuaba (Erythroxylum Catuaba) (Anemopegma mirandum)
Taste: light, slightly bitter
Energy: mildly relaxing

Catuaba is another plant with a long history in herbal medicine as an aphrodisiac. The Tupi Indians in Brazil first discovered the qualities of the plant, and over the last centuries, they have composed many songs praising its wonders. There is a saying which goes, "Until a father reaches 60, the son is his; after that the son is catuaba's." This refers to the dwindling vitality and fertility of men as they age.

If a man is over 60 years old and still manages to impregnate his lover the credit often goes to the power of catuaba. In Brazilian herbal medicine today, catuaba is considered a central nervous system stimulant with aphrodisiac properties used for sexual impotency, agitation, nervousness, poor memory or forgetfulness, and sexual weakness.

Making a tea of catuaba provides a relaxing effect whose flavor reminds me of cinnamon and pau d'arco.

Rose (Rosa Centifolia, Gallica, and Damascena are the most common varieties)
Taste: sweet and floral
Energetic: cooling

Rose has long been a symbol of love. Often given in grand bouquets or left on pillows after a night of passion, this aromatic flower has an unmistakable meaning. The medicinal properties show a strong affinity for the blood.

The essential oil of rose has been shown in studies to relax the nervous system and calm the mind. Rose is for the heart, physically and energetically, the center of love, whether that is love for one person or Universal love.

Rose oil helps love energy to radiate out. I like to include rose in most aphrodisiac formulas for its energetic ability to open the heart.

Vanilla (Vanilla planifolia)

Taste: sweet and aromatic

Energetic: neutral

In the 1700s physicians and alchemists recommended vanilla in a tea or alcohol extract to maintain male potency. In the 1800s, Dr. John King advised in the *American Dispensatory* that one should use vanilla to, "stimulate the sexual propensities."

The scent and flavor of vanilla is believed to increase lust. The long phallic shape of the seedpod is enough to classify it among the passionate foods. I love combining vanilla and chocolate together.

The seedpod contains what I call "love caviar," hundreds of tiny crunchy black seeds that are overwhelmingly yummy. I love seeing the tiny black flecks in sweet nut cream stuffed dates!

Cinnamon (Cinnamomum cassia)

Taste: sweet, spicy and slightly bitter

Energetic: warming

Cinnamon is great for male libido!! Herbalist James Duke researched that the smell of cinnamon in hot cinnamon buns stimulated blood flow to the penis. Cinnamon creates a warming action as well as an increase in circulation that can help treat sexual impotence.

Increasing the blood flow in the body means increasing the blood flow to the penis!! The flavor is so sweet and spicy that I find it to be a wonderful addition in almost any recipe, from warming beverages to chocolate balls.

Ginger (Zingiber officinale)

Taste: spicy and floral

Energetic: warming, stimulating

There is a lot of scientific evidence that supports ginger's wide range of medicinal actions. Ginger has been shown in research to increase sperm count & motility. Ginger increases circulation and brings warmth to the extremities.

In Chinese herbal medicine ginger warms the energy channels of the body.

A wonderful natural body deodorizer, ginger helps your sweat and secretions smell sweet. I find adding a pinch of ginger powder brings a gentle warmth and subtle spiciness to an aphrodisiac recipe that can increase the effects of the other herbs.

Cardamom (Elettaria cardamomum)
Taste: pungent and spicy
Energetic: warming

Cleopatra was known to bathe in cardamom for its sensual influence and aphrodisiac effects. The spice has a mild stimulating effect. It can be a wonderful addition to fruit dishes and chocolate spiced drinks. Check out the "lover's chai" recipe if you really want to "spice" it up!

Garlic (Allium sativum)
Taste: spicy, pungent, overpowering
Energetic: heating

Garlic has a long list of traditional uses as well as modern scientific research that point to many medicinal benefits, from heart disease to fungal infections. Its history as a spice of love is one of denial more than indulgence for the 'heat' in garlic is said to stir sexual desires.

Monks and other celibate spiritual practitioners have eliminated this culinary yumminess from their diet to lesson sexual desire. Also known as the "stinking rose," I recommend that you and your partner share it together or it might have the opposite effect; garlic breath isn't so sexy!

Ashwagandha (Withania somnifera)
Taste: slightly bitter, smooth; similar to ginseng
Energetic: warming

Ashwagandha is an herb that is extensively used, in Ayurveda, the traditional health care system in India, as a tonic and for its adaptogenic properties.

Historically, ashwagandha root has also been used for its sex-enhancing properties. It is a powerful overall tonic for greater vitality and longevity.

Ashwagandha enhances virility especially for men. It is beneficial for the treatment of involuntary ejaculation or drooling of semen without any sexual event/erection/orgasm.

In Indian herbal medicine this plant is used by both men and women to build life force and vitality. Ashwagandha builds efficacy over time so I recommend using it daily in tonic recipes.

American Ginseng (Panax quinquefolium)
Taste: bitter, pungent, earthy
Energetic: cooling

Ginseng is known for its stimulant properties as an aphrodisiac, especially in the East. Over time it improves the sexual function of both men and women and is used in the treatment of impotence and infertility.

A powerful adaptogen that helps the body deal with stress, I have found it to be a very effective way for men to increase their sexual vigor and stamina. Even a single dose before lovemaking goes a long way!

Kava Kava (Piper methysticum)
Taste: mild, numbing, bitter
Energetic: relaxing

Kava kava is known in Hawaii as the "anti-shyness" herb. One of the many amazing benefits of kava is that it relaxes without creating drowsiness, putting us in a more open and comfortable state that is quite conducive to both initiating and engaging with a lover.

Kava can increase a sense of euphoria while helping maintain our common sense, unlike alcohol. I like to brew kava in coconut milk, in the traditional style of the Polynesian culture. The fat in coconut milk is ideal for releasing the medicinal properties and making them available to you.

Kava has a numbing and tingling effect when the extract is rubbed on the external sexual organs. Don't go crazy here, less is more; you don't want to tingle too much! Trust me I figured that one out the hard way!

Horny Goat Weed (Epimedium grandiflorum)
Taste: mild, light flavor; similar to green tea with less bitterness
Energetic: warming

Horny goat weed is a traditional botanical medicine from China and Japan. It stimulates sexual activity in both men and women, increases sperm production, stimulates the sensory nerves, and increases sexual desire. In addition, research has shown that horny goat weed has anti-fatigue effects and helps prevents adrenal exhaustion.

Horny goat weed can increase energy levels or reduce stress depending on the needs of the body. As a tea it makes a light pleasant beverage. After 20 minutes of drinking the tea I find lightness in energy and a smooth, relaxed feeling. Drunken daily for several weeks, horny goat weed tea can dramatically improve the desire for sexual intimacy in both men and women.

Cayenne (Capsicum annum)
Taste: spicy
Energetic: hot, cooling in large doses due to increase in perspiration

Cayenne increases circulation and the pulse rate. It is a stimulant and has an irritant effect on the reproductive area. It stimulates nerve endings and releases endorphins which can give you a natural high.

I find it extremely helpful in recipes as a way of spreading the other herbs around the body by increasing circulation.

Rhodiola (Rhodiola rosea)
Taste: slightly floral and chocolaty
Energetic: neutral

Rhodiola has been frequently used in Viking folk medicine to increase physical strength and endurance and to promote fertility and longevity. It is presently used as an adaptogenic tonic to treat depression and fatigue. Rhodiola has been used to treat sexual disorders such as premature ejaculation and erectile dysfunction, while promoting fertility.

The root was often used in European folk love potions. From a 13th century myth comes the tale of a Ukrainian prince whose reputation was on par with Casanova. This prince, Danila Galitsky, was believed to have used rhodiola as an aphrodisiac. I find the smoky chocolate rose flavor to be an amazing alchemical bonus! I often include this plant in chocolate formulas because it will enhance the flavor!

Cubeb berries (Piper cubeba)
Taste: bitter, peppery (flavor)
Energetic: warming

One Thousand and One Nights, a Persian collection of folk tales, recommends cubeb berries as a remedy for infertility. A paste of the berries was used externally by Unani Physicians on the male and female genitals to intensify sexual pleasure.

Unani medicine is very close to Ayurveda but heavily influenced by Islam rather than Hinduism. Some traditional herbalists have used cubeb for its ability to warm and increase internal heat. Cubeb is popular among many Arabic medical texts for increasing desire and the treatment of gonorrhea. I love how nature works! The cause of your increased passion and the potential subsequent effects can be treated with the same plant!

Chocolate (Theobroma cacao)
Taste: bitter, smooth and rich
Energetic: heating

Chocolate has a long history dating back 5,000 years. Theobroma cacao, "Food of the Gods", was used as money and medicine, honored as a divine healing food it was used in ritualistic celebration. Raw chocolate is one of the greatest sources of magnesium. The high magnesium and antioxidant levels in chocolate help maintain blood pressure and support the heart directly; chocolate really does "open the heart"!

Raw chocolate is high in theobromine, a gentle nervous system stimulant. Phenylethylamine (PEA) and serotonin are also found in cacao!!! PEA is dubbed the "love chemical" due to its increase in the body when we fall in love.

When we are sexually aroused our brain releases PEA, peaking at orgasm. Chocolate keeps PEA levels high, even when not in love... hmmmm... no wonder women turn to chocolate so much... it truly is a comfort food!

Chocolate contains anandamide and anandamide inhibitors, which prevent the body from metabolizing it too quickly, elongating its effect in the body. Anandamide is released by the body when we are feeling great! Cacao (chocolate) contains tryptophan, an essential amino acid responsible for enhancing mood. The presence of all these mood elevating chemicals explains the aphrodisiac and addictive effects! Besides all the amazing effects, chocolate's flavor alone makes it worthy of its place as one of the most beloved aphrodisiacs.

Shatavari (Asparagus racemosus)
Taste: sweet, bitter, earthy
Energetic: cooling and calming

In Ayurveda Shatavari is considered the "Queen of Herbs" for women's health; the name translates to "A women with a hundred husbands." (Hmmm) Wonder why? It is used to treat all aspects of the female reproductive system and it is also known in traditional herbal medicine for its aphrodisiac properties when used over a period of time.

An excellent tonic herb for both men and women since it can nourish the blood, calm the nerves and build muscle tissue. It calms and stabilizes the emotions of the heart, promoting love and devotion. I like to use it in powder form by adding it to honey and chocolate as a tasty way of taking my daily "medicine."

Stinging Nettle (Urtica dioica)
Taste: green, grassy, light
Energetic: cooling

Nettle is an excellent tea herb and a must in any tonic formula. It nourishes and energizes the endocrine glands and strengthens the nervous system. Nettle is a skin irritant if you touch the stinging leaves which then cause an increase of circulation to that area. The dried or fresh leaf in tea has a wonderful healing effect on the female reproductive system.

Stinging nettle has been used to tone the walls of the uterus, rehydrate dry vaginal walls and relieve night sweats and hot flashes. Okay, I had to include this fact for anyone out there daring enough, so if S&M is your thing then this might be for you!

There was a practice of nettle flagellation where you whip your naked partner, particularly in the genital region, with fresh nettles until erection or lust occurs. For the rest of you, drinking nettle tea, high in calcium, magnesium, potassium, iron and vitamins A, C and E, can provide essential nutrition that may be key to increasing your sexual desire!

Nutmeg (Myristica fragrans)
Taste: spicy
Energetic: stimulating and warming

Nutmeg is wonderfully aromatic and spicy! It is believed to impart strength and enhance sexual ability. Nutmeg is a strong stimulant/inebriant used in love magic.

The active ingredient, myristicin, is the base of MDA or Ecstasy, the "love drug." Large quantities have been used to achieve altered states but with some unpleasant side effects, mostly nausea. I find nutmeg to be more effective as an aphrodisiac when used sparingly as a spice in recipes.

Saffron (Crocus sativus)
Taste: slightly bitter, aromatic, earthy
Energetic: hot and dry

Citizens of the Roman Empire sought saffron as a healing herb and aphrodisiac. The wealthiest Romans would sprinkle their marriage beds with saffron to christen a prosperous union.

Saffron has stimulating properties on the erogenous zones. A lovely addition to chocolate, saffron warms the whole body, especially the heart. For women, saffron stimulates sexual desire, strengthens the uterus and treats menstrual problems. Some experimenters claim the essential oil can evoke long, distinctive orgasms. In high doses saffron oil is toxic – so be careful!

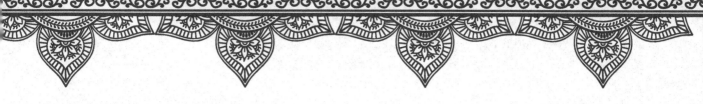

CHAPTER 7

SUPER FOODS

In the past super foods may have been considered aphrodisiacs because they provided a richly expansive range of nutrients when overall nutrition was poor. Undernourishment was a frequent battle before there were grocery stores that provide a rainbow of choices. Super foods are full of vitamins, minerals, amino acids and enzymes that can help increase libido all on their own. Over all health may be better today but because of the fast food industry and the availability of quick, easy snack foods, most people are overeating and not receiving the right vitamins to sustain them never mind reach optimal performance. Super foods can offer that extra jolt of energy by providing diverse nutrients that our modern diet may be lacking.

My favorite foods that I incorporate into formulas and bedside dishes are often chosen for their nutrient content. These foods are often times labeled as "super foods." Combining them with powerful plants will alchemically increase the potency of the aphrodisiac.

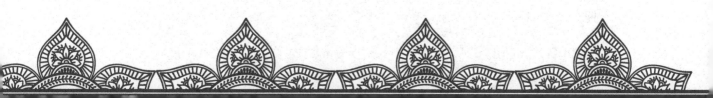

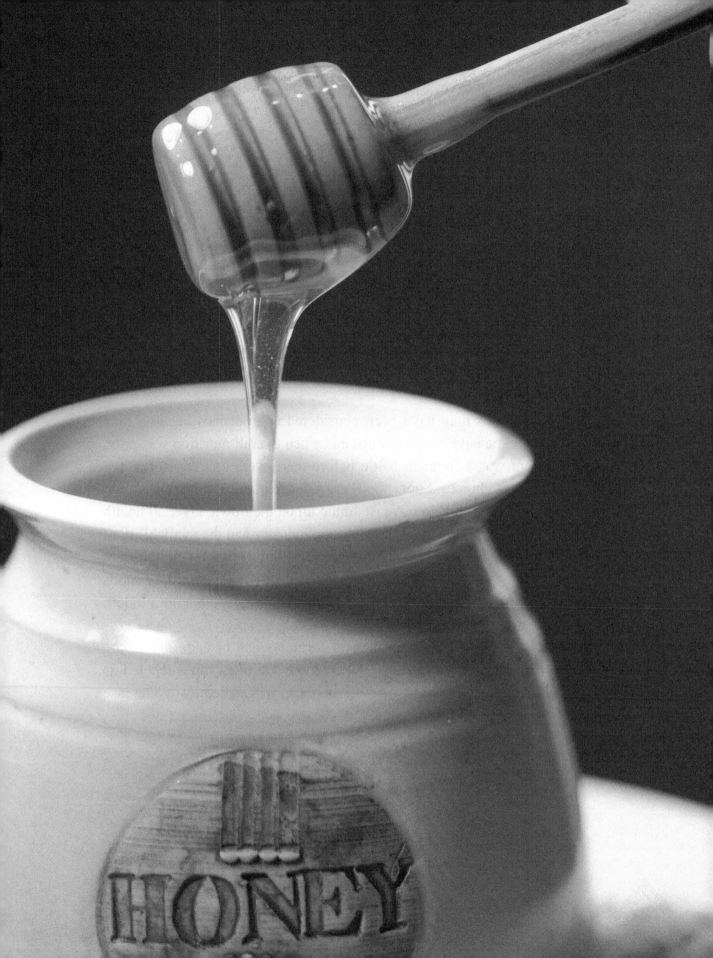

Bee pollen

Bee pollen has a warming sweetness and is capable of providing extreme amounts of energy and vitality. Literally the sex of the flowers, pollen inspires sensuality by its very nature. Taken daily, it can build the body with its rich array of vitamins and nutrients. Start off with a small dose, people with seasonal allergies may be sensitive! In the long run daily doses of local bee pollen can help cure those yearly allergies!

Royal Jelly

The only bee in a hive that is allowed to eat the royal jelly produced in honey making is the Queen. She is also the only one who is capable of fertility, and, she lives longer than any other bee. Is it a coincidence? Rich in B vitamins and enzymes, royal jelly is the best super food for inspiring fertility. In most health food stores it comes in honey and is easy to add to most recipes.

Raw honey

Raw Honey is unheated and unfiltered, leaving the abundant enzymes, vitamins and minerals naturally present intact. The bees collect nectar from flowers and combine it with their saliva to make honey. They also collect plant resins to combine with their saliva to form propolis, an antibacterial "glue" they use to seal and protect the honey in the hives.

Raw honey often has traces of propolis and pollen in its list of nutrients, making it a powerful healing aid. Due to its antibacterial nature honey was a natural preservative for many medicines in Egyptian times including cures for sterility and impotence.

Medieval seducers offered their partners mead, a fermented drink made from honey. It is an old German custom for newlyweds to drink this sweet fermented beverage for one month after the wedding to promote fertility. This time was called the honey month, later coined the honeymoon!

Almonds

Almonds are known for their intoxicating aroma and have been used in soaps and body lotions to excite the senses. Some traditions used almonds to treat premature ejaculation in men. They are a rich source of vitamins and healthy fats that can nourish a depleted body. A daily tonic from Ayurvedic medicine suggests 10 soaked, peeled almonds with 3 dates every morning. I like to use raw almond butter in some recipes for the nourishing qualities and delicious flavor.

Pine nuts

Pine nuts have been used to stimulate the libido since medieval times. They are rich in zinc, a key mineral necessary to maintain male potency. I like to use powdered nuts as a base in a lot of my recipes, especially the soft fatty ones like cashew, macadamia and pine nuts. My first choice is usually pine nuts since they supply aphrodisiac qualities all on their own!

Raw chocolate

Even though I already listed chocolate in the herb section I wanted to include it here with the super foods. Full of vitamins, minerals, antioxidants and stimulants, chocolate has a long reputation for stimulating the sexual senses.

Blue green algae

There is something about including the rich green color in my concoctions that inspires me but blue green algae isn't just a wonderful way to add color to a recipe. It is rich in trace minerals, which help other vitamins and enzymes to perform their various functions in the body.

Blue green algae is full of fortifying nutrients like essential amino acids that cannot be manufactured by the body yet are vital to health and sexual functioning, like maintaining an erection. The wonderful green color I love so much is due to the high chlorophyll content. Chlorophyll is very similar to our own human blood. This "plant blood" functions in the plant the way our human blood circulates for us.

Consuming blue green algae is a fantastic way to support the circulation of oxygen throughout the body. And as we have learned, the more oxygen and blood flow in the body, the more in the genitals!!!!

Pumpkin seeds

Pumpkin seeds are high in zinc, an essential nutrient for men's sexual health. Raw pumpkin seeds are also a source of magnesium, iron, phosphorus, calcium, vitamin A, and vitamin B. These nutrients are necessary in the healthy production of sex hormones.

Eating a handful of pumpkin seeds daily may help prevent impotence! Their essential fatty acids are excellent for nourishing both men and women. One easy way I sneak them into chocolate recipes is to roll/dust the finished product in ground pumpkin seed flour. It gives a nice decorative touch while packing in the nutrients!

Chia seeds

The word chia is derived from the Mayan language, meaning "strength." I read that Aztec warriors relied on chia seeds to boost energy and increase stamina. They are high in fiber and omega 3's. I like to include it in recipes as an endurance enhancing super food. It swells up and gets gooey if you add it to water. My preferred use is mixed in with nuts and chocolate.

Goji berries

These small dried red fruits are full of nutrients. Rich in vitamins, minerals, amino acids and anti-oxidants the list of health benefits range from anti-aging to improved eyesight.

In China, the goji is called "happy berry", in part due to its history as an aphrodisiac tonic for male infertility and sexual weakness. They are very tasty and blend well with raw chocolate. I discovered, while trying to powder them, if I added one teaspoon of cacao powder in the grinder they wouldn't stick in one clump. It makes it so much easier to include their lovely flavor in recipes this way!

Acai fruit

This purple berry comes from the rain forests of the Amazon. Acai berries have high levels of antioxidants, essential amino acids and fatty acids. They are rich in antioxidants that are capable of slowing down aging. Acai berries share a common feel good chemical with chocolate, the stimulate theobromine.

The acai fruit was traditionally consumed by mixing the pulp of the fruit with Guarana seed. The result was an energizing super power concoction! Although the berry itself isn't sweet, the natural chocolate berry flavor blended with a sweetener becomes a strange new sensation to crave!

Pineapple

Fresh pineapple fruit juice has traditionally been used for its healing affect on the digestive system. In homeopathy it is a remedy for treating impotence.

Drink a small glass daily to promote the energies of love and make the sexual secretions taste sweeter! I like to dip the rim of an empty glass in raw honey and then in dried coconut before serving a cup of chilled pineapple juice. Delicious sticky yumminess!

Durian fruit

Ahhh durian, "the king of fruits!" Before I begin to worship this amazing fruit I must provide a disclaimer so that you are prepared for your first meeting: most people don't like durian at first. They are usually turned off by the smell and then skeptical to taste it. With a strong pungent garlicky odor, this spiky fruit does everything in its power to turn people off… that is until they have tasted it.

Often after several trials they become almost feverishly passionate for this creamy sweet fruit. The occasional lucky durian fanatic enjoys its flavor on the first trial. Once you're hooked, watch out! Some clinical studies have shown that the chemical composition of durian can create a similar reaction as a drug induced state and is possibly addictive!

Durian is full of tryptophan, that wonderfully relaxing chemical. After living in Thailand for several years and frequently visiting Malaysia, I can vouch for the incredible effects of durian on my desire and libido. Durian is very heating to the body and makes me feel lustful and restless only thirty minutes after eating! The local Thai women in the market near my house used to laugh and tell me to feed it to my boyfriend to have good "boom boom!"

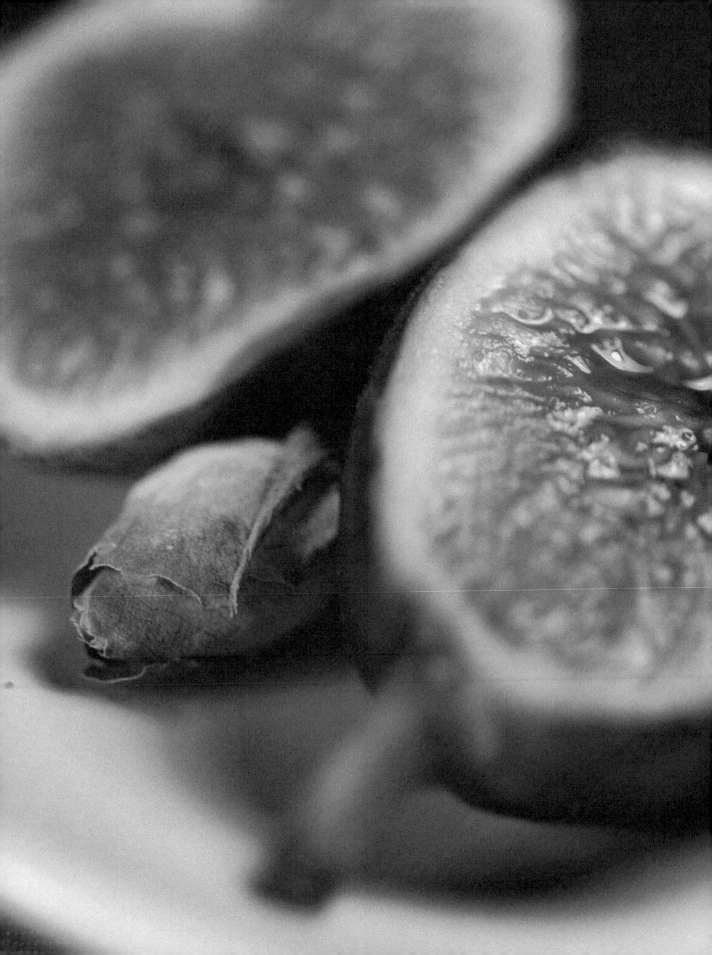

CHAPTER 8

FOODS CONSIDERED APHRODISIAC DUE TO PHALLIC OR YONI SHAPES

Some foods have a long historical reputation for increasing desire and passion, like oysters and caviar. Others are used for their physical resemblance to genitalia. One day, someone must have looked at a carrot and had related it to an erect penis. I can just imagine the random "Ah-Ha!" moment: "If it looks like a penis… hmmm… maybe it will… help my penis!?!"

Foods like asparagus, bananas and cucumbers have been used because of their resemblance to a rigid phallus. There are foods that inspire the female image of sensuality as well. For example, a fresh fig cut in half has an uncanny resemblance to the yoni, or vagina.

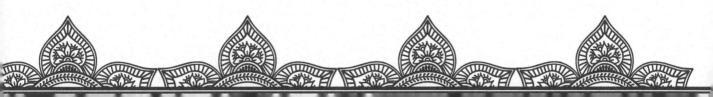

Asparagus

As a diuretic, asparagus stimulates the activity of the kidneys. In traditional Chinese herbal medicine the kidneys are the organ system responsible for sexual vitality and longevity. A traditional folk saying states that people who eat a lot of asparagus also have many lovers. The long penis shaped stalks are mighty suggestive to your lover across the table if you were to slowly nibble one down to your fingertips. Leave the fork aside, this vegetable is much sexier when eaten with the hands!

Cucumber

There isn't too much evidence on a chemical level that cucumbers affect the libido. I believe its reputation has more to do with its physical applications as a phallus than its medicinal properties, but think it worth mentioning anyway!

Aside from its phallic shape, the scent of cucumbers is believed to stimulate women by increasing blood flow to the vagina. There is a reason why there are so many jokes about women, cucumbers and masturbation.

I once had a set of playing cards that had the phrase "Why cucumbers are better than men…" on one side and a laughable answer on the other: "Because a cucumber will always stay hard!" Whether or not there is any truth to the claim of its aphrodisiac powers, cucumbers certainly have a reputation as a pleasure giving veggie.

Okra

Okra is penis shaped and filled with a sticky, gooey mucus. Is it hard to imagine why many cultures believe it to be an aphrodisiac? Okra is actually the fruit of the plant and a rich source of magnesium, iron, zinc and B vitamins. I have never been successful in creating a chocolate okra recipe, but I love it as a main course in a romantic meal!

Raspberries and strawberries

Raspberries and strawberries are perfect foods for hand feeding your lover. Both invite love and are described in erotic literature as "fruit nipples."

Strawberries have a lovely heart shape and luscious red color. They are high in antioxidants and vitamin C. Try dipping them in a herb-infused chocolate sauce!

Fresh fig

The fig is traditionally thought of as sexual stimulant. An open fig can be visually compared to the female sex organs. Referred to as the "fruit of the Goddess" by one of my friends I always feel sensual biting into a fresh juicy fig.

CHAPTER 9

WHAT IS ALCHEMY?

Alchemy can be simply defined as changing one thing into another. Many alchemists sought to discover the secret of turning base metals into gold. Alchemy is the ancient predecessor of chemistry. It has a reputation of mysticism and a feel for the esoteric. The goal of ancient alchemy was to achieve spiritual development by the mystical realization of the nature, behavior and transformation of certain substances and the energies within.

To me, alchemy is the art of transforming things into something completely different. The process of successful alchemical blending is more than correct measurements. It is everything: the mood of the alchemist, the environment, the vitality of the ingredients and the intention behind the act of creation. This final result of a unique and harmonious blend is a new complete product.

In another way we can look at lovemaking as the ultimate alchemical experience. Two separate bodies come together in harmony to create one new experience. The two bodies blend energy, hormones and secretions to produce a state of consciousness and physical pleasure that is a unique alchemical manifestation. This ultimate union, the merging of two people into one consciousness is often the goal of tantric lovemaking. Shiva and Shakti, the male and female energies, become one. The masculine and the feminine dissolve into one another and pure love abounds. Aphrodisiac plants can be used alchemically to facilitate this transformation when lovers hold this intention.

There are so many elements to consider when you decide to experiment with aphrodisiacs. There is the physical aspect, which takes into consideration the

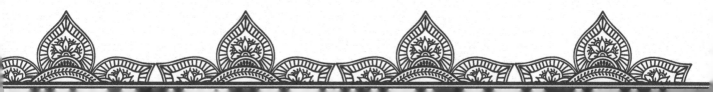

chemical components, the taste and the smell. The energetic aspects, which refers to the heating or cooling effects in the body, the level of activation on the subtle energetic planes and the exchange between the alchemist and the plant itself. Lastly there is the purely alchemical aspect of blending, using knowledge of the physical and energetic aspects, to draw out the fullest potential of each plant while creating a harmoniously balanced aphrodisiac.

Raw Chocolate

A good number of the recipes in this book include raw chocolate. Cacao, commonly called raw chocolate, is the uncooked, unroasted, unprocessed bean. Most conventional chocolate you buy in candy or eat in cakes and brownies has been roasted and processed. Nearly all types of chocolate found in stores are adulterated with large amounts of chemicals, fats and sugar. The majority of the vitamins, minerals and antioxidants are lost or significantly reduced by the roasting process.

Raw Chocolate (cacao)	vs.	Conventional Chocolate
• Uncooked, unprocessed • Higher in enzymes minerals, vitamins and stimulants that are lost when cooked		• Cacao beans are fermented and roasted before being processed into cocoa liquor, powder and unsweetened bricks • more likely to cause an allergic reaction • loss of some of the nutrient value from heating

As you can see, raw chocolate is generally healthier and it provides more vital life force, more energy. You can buy raw chocolate at most health food stores and online with raw food supply companies.

The making of conventional chocolate is an art form unto itself, involving many steps. Once the chocolatier has mixed all the ingredients they will take the chocolate through the conching process. Here a special machine is used to massage the chocolate in order to blend the ingredients together and make it smooth. Next comes tempering, a controlled heating and cooling process. Without tempering, the chocolate does not harden properly.

When making raw chocolate treats we skip these steps to avoid heating and destroying vital nutrients. My discovery and implementation of raw chocolate has been quite an experimental journey. I still desired the smooth creamy texture of conventional chocolate with my earthy uncooked cacao beans. Over time I learned little secrets and shared in some experiments with other raw chocolatiers until I was satisfied with the results. I am happy to pass them onto you!

Here is a list of some of the key chocolate making ingredients:

Raw cacao butter

Raw cacao butter is the true white chocolate. When cacao is cold pressed the oil is separated from the bean. This oil, cacao oil, is also known as cacao butter or coco butter in stores. Due to its high saturated fat content it is usually solid unless in a very hot climate. Saturated fats are typically solid at room temperature. After the oil is pressed out the rest of the bean is dried and made into cacao powder.

Raw coconut oil

Most coconut oil you buy in stores is highly refined. Raw coconut oil is cold pressed and full of healing properties. Best of all, the flavor is pure delight! Truly raw coconut oil smells fresh; as though we just cracked open a coconut while lying on some exotic beach.

Raw agave nectar

Agave nectar is a natural sweetener produced from the Tequila cactus. Its flavor is mild and very sweet, sweeter than sugar. The darker agave nectar has a slight metallic taste due to the higher mineral content.

Coconut sap sugar

One of the lowest glycemic natural sweeteners available, this delicious sugar is the collected sap from the flower bud of the coconut palm tree. The sap is cooked and air-dried into light brown crystals. I have discovered a simple way to make syrup from the crystals that blows my mind and taste buds! Take 1 cup of coconut sugar and add 2 tbs of boiling water. Stir until mostly smooth. Let it sit overnight to remove any granules or chunks and voila, sweet and smooth sap syrup!

Raw honey

Honey is a magical alchemical substance made from the nectar of flowers. When bees make honey it is stored in the waxy comb. Most honey makers heat the honeycomb and spin it through a filter to separate out the wax and resins. Raw honey has never been heated above a mild temperature, if it all, so the propolis and royal jelly are able to remain present in the honey. Raw honey has a rich flavor and tastes alive!

Now you can enjoy my time tested recipes and alchemical revelations with a better knowledge of what I believe to be one of the most amazing aphrodisiacs on the planet: raw cacao!

ALCHEMICAL CHOCOLATE MAKING

When using raw cacao, raw chocolate, I had to stumble through many boo boo's and mistakes until I discovered the perfect alchemical harmony. Here is a description, a journey into my discovery of working with raw cacao.

One of the first things I learned was how volatile the oil is when making chocolate. The state of the oil effects how well the other ingredients blend together. I like to use the raw cacao and raw coconut oils. They are saturated fats, which means that at cool temperatures they are solid and when heated they become liquid. The liquid form of the oil is better for making chocolate so that a perfect blending of fat and sweetener can occur.

Once the oil has liquefied, I add the sweetener (honey, agave, etc.). Blending them together at first seems futile, but after a couple minutes the two accept each other and become a beautiful thick, caramel-like sauce. The texture is smooth and the smell is chocolate bliss. Don't let the sauce sit for too long or the oil and the sweetener will separate again. There is only a small window of time for alchemical perfection. It is this consistency that I find ideal for blending herbs and chocolate into a delicious edible treat.

Just as in traditional baking, I found that it was important to mix all the dry ingredients together first. Once all the powdered herbs, chocolate and nut flours have been placed in a bowl spend time gently mixing them together, with intention and inspiration. The physical blending of the ingredients is important so that when the liquid is added everything will already be mixed up in equal proportions and every bite will have a harmony of all the ingredients.

The energetic alchemy that happens as you mix the dry ingredients together is just as important as the physical. The thoughts and feelings you have as you mix are infusing the recipe. This is the time to focus on positive intention, pleasurable images, thoughts and desires into the bowl. I often draw sacred symbols into the dry mix while chanting yogic mantras or singing. The more genuine energy I bring to the aphrodisiac making experience, the more genuine energy goes into the final product. I have shared recipes with friends and often heard feedback that their aphrodisiac results didn't seem as powerful as mine. Upon investigation, I discovered that they had dismissed the importance of setting a positive, loving mood and infusing the kitchen experience with intention and energy. Half of the magic and success of aphrodisiacs is in the energetic alchemy!

Alchemical Secrets

If you have ever eaten out at a restaurant that really impressed you I guarantee that if you asked the chef she would confess her love of food and cooking. When someone loves to cook you can taste it. It is the ultimate secret ingredient. You may not associate good food with a good attitude but your deeper subconscious does.

The amazing studies Masaru Emoto did on water crystals are perfect example of the power our thoughts and words carry. Mr. Emoto conducted experiments that provided evidence that human vibrational energy, thoughts and words, affect the molecular structure of water. He taped words onto glass jars filled with distilled water and then photographed the crystals that formed when the water was frozen. Positive words, like love and gratitude, created harmonious crystals of beauty, while negative ones, like hate, created chaos and mismatched shapes.

As you find yourself ready to play in the kitchen with these recipes take time to create a relaxed, happy, sensuous state. Cultivate a feeling of joy, have fun with the process! If you are rushing, distracted or uncentered that energy will become a part of your aphrodisiac creation, so be sure you have plenty of time and no distractions when you decide to play in the kitchen.

Setting your intention is extremely important for the alchemy of creating. My favorite intention is to worship the plants and other ingredients as divine gifts sent to help me open to love. I visualize myself as a servant of the divine and offer up all of my actions and their effects to the idea of supreme love, bliss and universal harmony for all beings everywhere.

Before you begin I recommend you stand in your kitchen and pause for a moment. Close your eyes and with all of your ingredients laid out on the counter offer your efforts up to something greater... Love! Here is a prayer I like to use:

"May these herbs and spices serve the highest purpose of all beings who consume them by increasing the flow of energy and grace. I have faith with all my heart that these sacred plants will help increase love, light and healing. May my hands infuse and charge this alchemical manifestation with love and pure intention for the most sacred and cosmic orgasmic experience."

Feel free to create your own prayer of intention, just be sure that it represents your truest intention and energy.

Alchemical Tips and Must Do's for Blissful Results!!!

Here are some tips for cultivating a harmonious alchemical experience:

- When making a chocolate recipe always include a few granules of salt or as much as a pinch depending on the formula. The salt shouldn't be noticeable in the flavor. The presence provides a subtle awakening of the tongue. Both salt and sugar stimulate the taste buds and create the sensation of flavor. Using a good quality salt with trace minerals is a key to alchemy. My theory is that the charge of the salt and the minerals affect the absorption and distribution of the main ingredients. It feels as though the essence of the salt helps drive the aphrodisiacs deeper into the body.

- If we are going to use cacao powder in a recipe, it is good to use a little cacao butter too. When the bean was whole both elements existed together. Some students have asked, "Why not just powder the bean and use it?" You can, and it is a wonderful option. But to use the pressed powder and butter creates a very unique texture that is unavailable with the ground whole bean. After pressing the oil out and processing the bean we get two completely different substances: Cacao powder and Cacao butter. By putting them back together again in a recipe you are completing the energy bond, but in a new alchemical way. The same ingredients processed differently create a different result. This is alchemy!!!

- Always, always, ALWAYS use your hands in the final mixing/blending!!! There is a natural tempering of the chocolate as it receives heat from your hands. Your hands are charged with energy and by using them in the mixing process you help infuse the plants with more healing potential. The sensuality of touching the chocolate and the herbs as they run through your hands is also very powerful; the more sensuous you feel while mixing the more sensuality goes into the product. In fact, I love to take my time mixing and allow the feeling of the herbs and foods to inspire a sense of pleasure and desire. As my passion builds, the aphrodisiac I am making becomes even more infused and powerful.

- Playing sensual music in the background is very helpful. Something that inspires you to visualize, dance, sway your hips or sing out loud. Create the mood you wish to arouse with the aphrodisiac!

- Use ceramic, wood or glass for mixing and stirring the ingredients. The resonance of natural materials is cleaner than those of aluminum, non-stick, tin or plastic.

- Consider preparing your alchemical creations nude! Or wear some sexy lingerie or a beautiful sarong. The more you can do to create a sensuous state of being, the more that energy goes into your recipes!

- A relationship with your alchemical materials is essential in pleasuring the taste buds! Take time to know your spices! I suggest spending time with them, sit down and smell each one. One by one, smell and then taste. Take note of each one's flavor. Is it strong and pungent? Light and sweet? Bitter? Mild? I love cardamom and tend to use it in a lot of recipes but it wasn't until I spent time with the spice that I learned how to use it. It is very strong and overpowering, and a little too much can ruin the flavor of a recipe. With an awareness of its taste, I know how to use it sparingly, to create a subtle spicy note in the right recipes. Enjoy getting to know your culinary companions!

— ଓ —

CHAPTER 10

RECIPES

Time for Tantalizing Taste buds!

TONICS

Now you understand that there are several ways to increase passion and desire with herbs. The following recipes are considered tonic formulas because they are designed to rejuvenate and tone the body by regulating and normalizing hormonal function and circulation. They build vitality with super-absorbable nutrients. Tonics are slow acting formulas, but when consumed over a period of time they can produce remarkable effects. We all want the" easy one time only" quick fix, but if you are really serious about building the body up to handle extreme passion then you will appreciate the use of tonics.

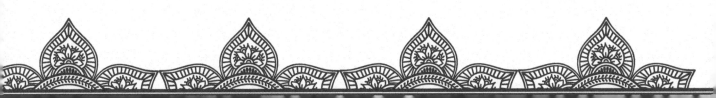

PINE NUT NIGHTS

The Perfumed Garden, an ancient Arabic love manual, contains many references to pine nuts including this prescription to restore a man's sexual vigor: "A glass of thick honey plus 20 almonds and 100 pine nuts repeated for three nights."

—❃—

OJAS BREAKFAST

Taken from my Ayurvedic doctor's recommendation for rebuilding ojas every morning, this simple recipe can help strengthen the body. Ojas, translated from Sanskrit, means vigor. According to Ayurvedic medicine it is the essential energy of the body. For building vital life force soak 10 almonds overnight and in the morning peel off the brown skin. Eat these almonds with 2-3 dates first thing for breakfast.

—❃—

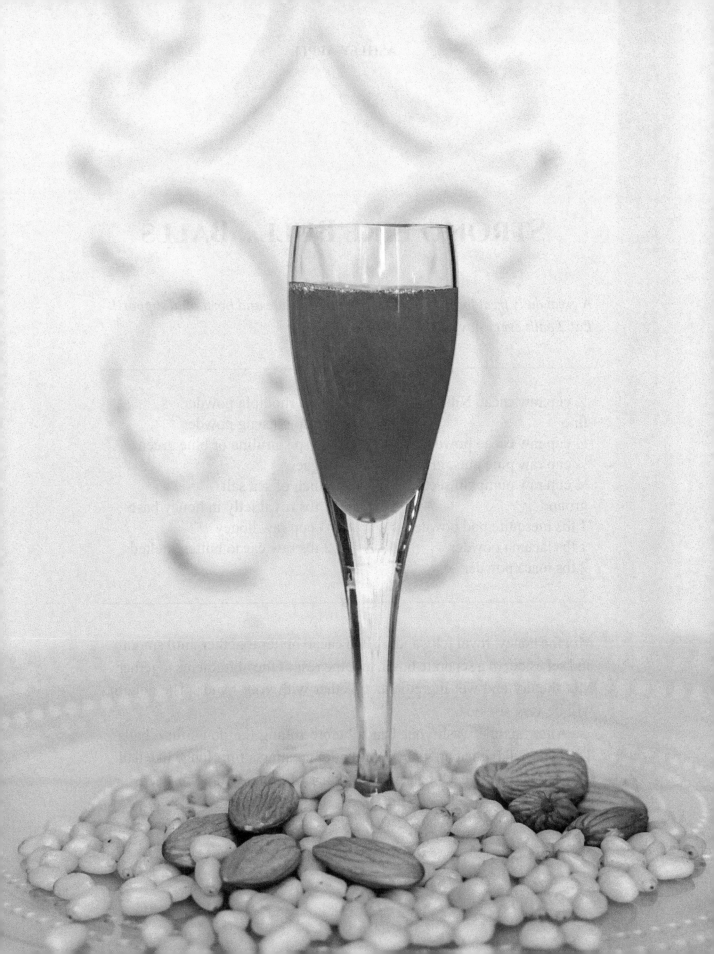

Strong Like Bull... Balls

A great daily treat for men to indulge in for prostate and hormonal support! Eat 2 balls every day for several weeks.

ᴄꙅ

¼ cup raw cacao Nibs, ground fine
½ cup raw cacao powder
⅛ cup raw pine nuts, ground
⅛ cup raw pumpkin seeds, ground
1 tbs mesquite pod powder
1 tbs lacuma powder
2 tbs maca powder

1 tsp rhodiola powder
½ tsp ginseng powder
½ tsp spirulina or blue green algae
pinch of sea salt
1 tbs royal jelly in honey base
¼ cup raw honey
2 tbs raw cacao butter, melted

ᴄꙅ

Mix the honey, royal jelly and melted cacao butter together until smooth and set aside. In a separate bowl, mix the rest of the ingredients together. Mix the dry and wet ingredients together with your hands. The dough will be very sticky.

After mixing, wash your hands before rolling the dough into balls. The balls will harden up in the refrigerator creating a firm fudge like ball.

Optional: Roll each ball into a mixture of ground pumpkin seeds or coconut flakes.

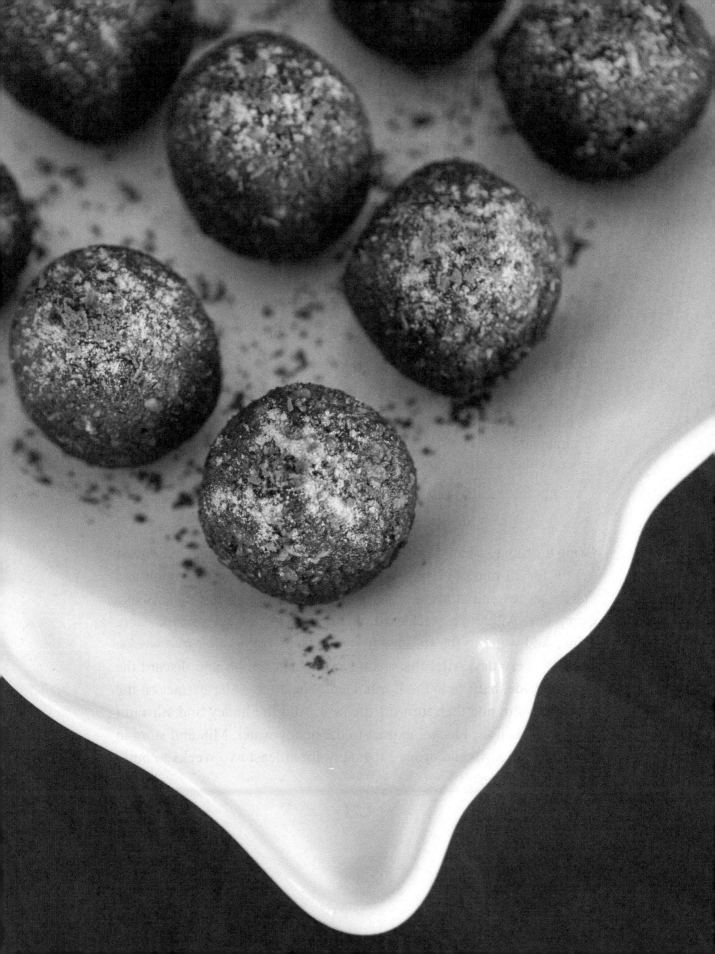

VIRA ELIXIR

This delicious elixir is ideal for men who want to increase their vitality, virility and stamina. This tonic takes several weeks to prepare.

½ cup muira puma
½ cup catuaba
2 cinnamon sticks
½ cup cubeb berries

7 cups rum
7 cups spring/filtered water
4 cups raw honey

Bring the rum to a light simmer in a pot and add the muira puma. Simmer gently for 20 minutes covered. Cool. Add the catuaba, cinnamon and cubeb berries and store in a glass jar with lid for two weeks. Shake every day. After two weeks, strain the alcohol extract off and store aside. Add water to the strained herb and steep for another two weeks, shaking every day. After the second two weeks, strain and discard the herbs outside, back onto the Earth. Gently heat the water extract on the stove to warm and then turn off the heat. Add the honey and stir until dissolved. Add the alcohol extract to the honey water. Mix and store in a glass jar. Men should drink 2 tbs daily for at least two weeks to build vitality and potency!

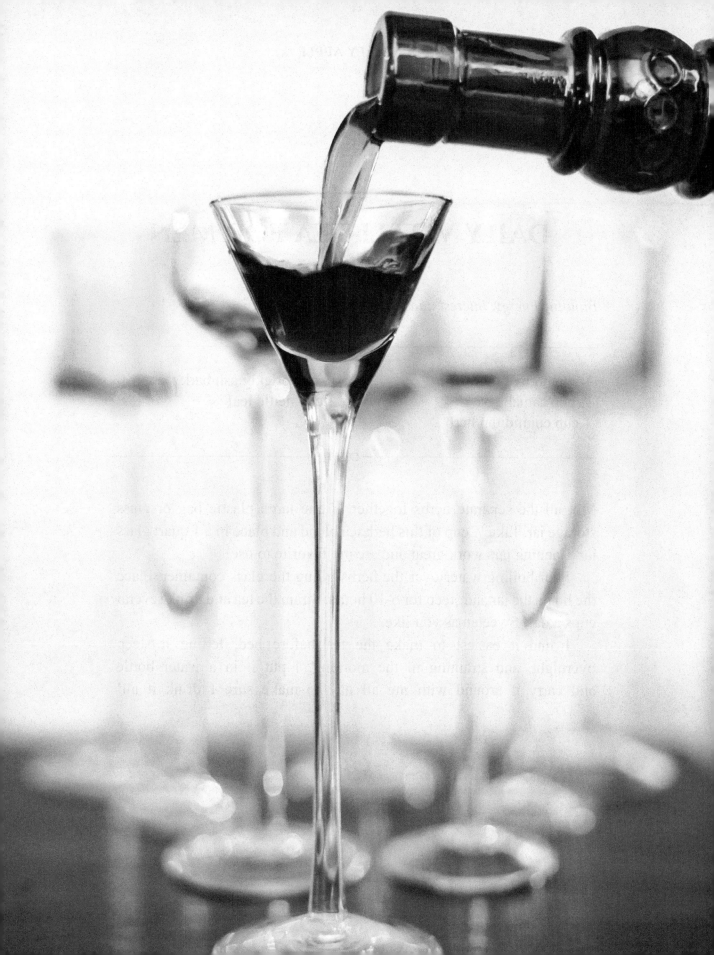

DAILY VITALI-TEA FOR MEN

Building Energy, Interest and Stamina

---

1 cup horny goat weed
½ cup catuaba bark
1 cup epimidium herb

½ cup prickly ash bark
1 cup nettle leaf

Mix all the separate herbs together in one large plastic bag or glass storage jar. Take ½ cup of this herb tea blend and place in a 1 quart glass jar. Canning jars work great and are my favorite to use!

Pour boiling water over the herbs filling the glass container. Place the lid on the jar and steep for 6-10 hours. Strain the tea and drink several cups a day. Sweeten as you like.

I find it easiest to make the tea before bed, letting it steep overnight, and straining in the morning. I put it in a water bottle and carry it around with me all day to make sure I drink it all!

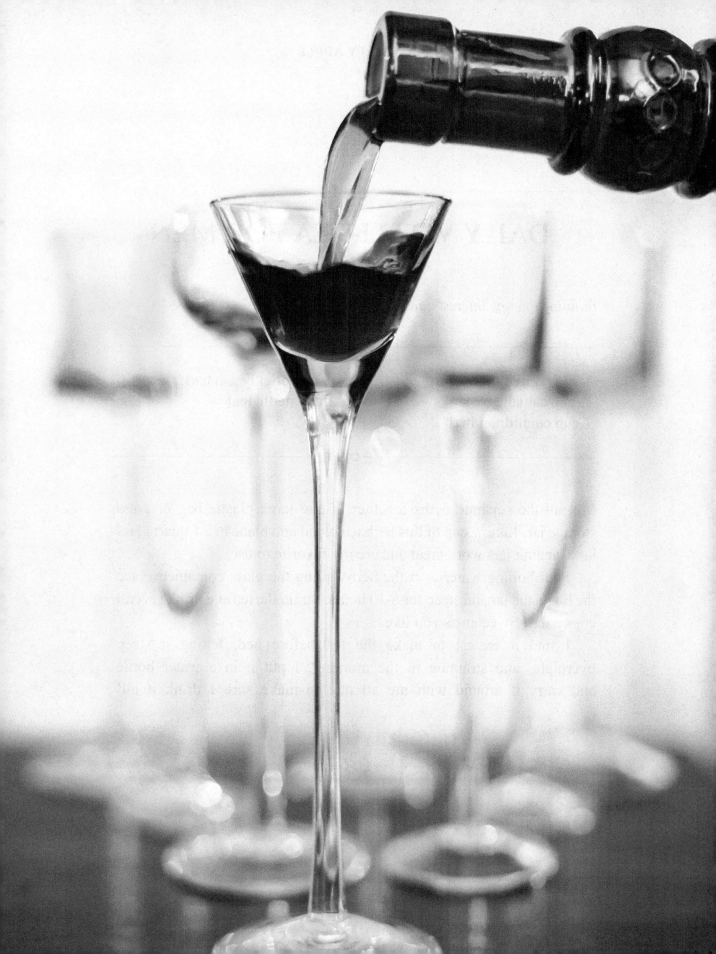

DAILY VITALI-TEA FOR MEN

Building Energy, Interest and Stamina

---

1 cup horny goat weed   ½ cup prickly ash bark
½ cup catuaba bark   1 cup nettle leaf
1 cup epimidium herb

Mix all the separate herbs together in one large plastic bag or glass storage jar. Take ½ cup of this herb tea blend and place in a 1 quart glass jar. Canning jars work great and are my favorite to use!

Pour boiling water over the herbs filling the glass container. Place the lid on the jar and steep for 6-10 hours. Strain the tea and drink several cups a day. Sweeten as you like.

I find it easiest to make the tea before bed, letting it steep overnight, and straining in the morning. I put it in a water bottle and carry it around with me all day to make sure I drink it all!

DAILY VITALI-TEA FOR WOMEN

A warming tonic for the female reproductive and hormonal system

½ cup damiana Leaf
1 cup raspberry Leaf
½ cup dried ginger root chunks

½ cup cinnamon bark, chopped
up in small chunks

Mix all the separate herbs together in one large plastic bag or glass storage jar.

Take ½ cup of this herb tea blend and place in a 1 quart glass jar. Canning jars work great and are my favorite to use! Pour boiling water over the herbs filling the glass container. Place the lid on the jar and steep for 6-10 hours.

Strain the tea and drink several cups a day. Sweeten as you like.

I find it easiest to make the tea before bed, letting it steep overnight, and straining in the morning. I put it in a water bottle and carry it around with me all day to make sure I drink it all!

DAILY SMOOTHIE TONIC POWDERS

Hormone regulating for men and women

These powdered herb formulas can be added to a daily smoothie as a tasty way of consuming aphrodisiac tonics. Use your favorite protein powder, or fruit smoothie recipe! A basic smoothie base is milk, dairy, soy or rice, fresh fruit like bananas and ice.

HORMONE SUPPORT

─────────────────────── ❧ ───────────────────────

½ cup maca powder   ½ cup tbs lacuma powder
½ cup tbs Suma powder   ½ cup tbs rhodiola powder

─────────────────────── ❧ ───────────────────────

Add all the herbs together in a jar or plastic bag and mix well. Add 1tbs of the mixed powders to your favorite smoothie base every day to build and support the body.

─ ❧ ─

VITALITY SMOOTHIE

½ cup Ashwagandha powder
½ cup tbs Suma powder

3 tbs ginseng powder

Add all the herbs together in a jar or plastic bag and mix well. Add 1tbs of the mixed powders to your favorite smoothie base every day to build and support the body.

"RIGHT NOW BABY!!!"

Believe it or not, there are amazing aphrodisiacs that can produce almost immediate effects. Most of these herbs have a dramatic effect on the nervous system, either immediately relaxing or immediately stimulating the physical body. Eat these recipes on a light or empty stomach to feel the most dramatic effects. These "ready right now" recipes are ideal for special one night plans and romantic rendezvous.

If you or your partner is experiencing decreased interest or has physical problems, these recipes may not be the long term solution. Head back to tonics and try out some of those formulas for a period of time. For the healthy couples that simply desire a spicy mood, a little extra oomph or a jolt of superhero energy to last the night, forge forward into my time-tested recipes for magical passionate awakenings.

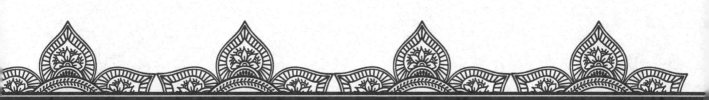

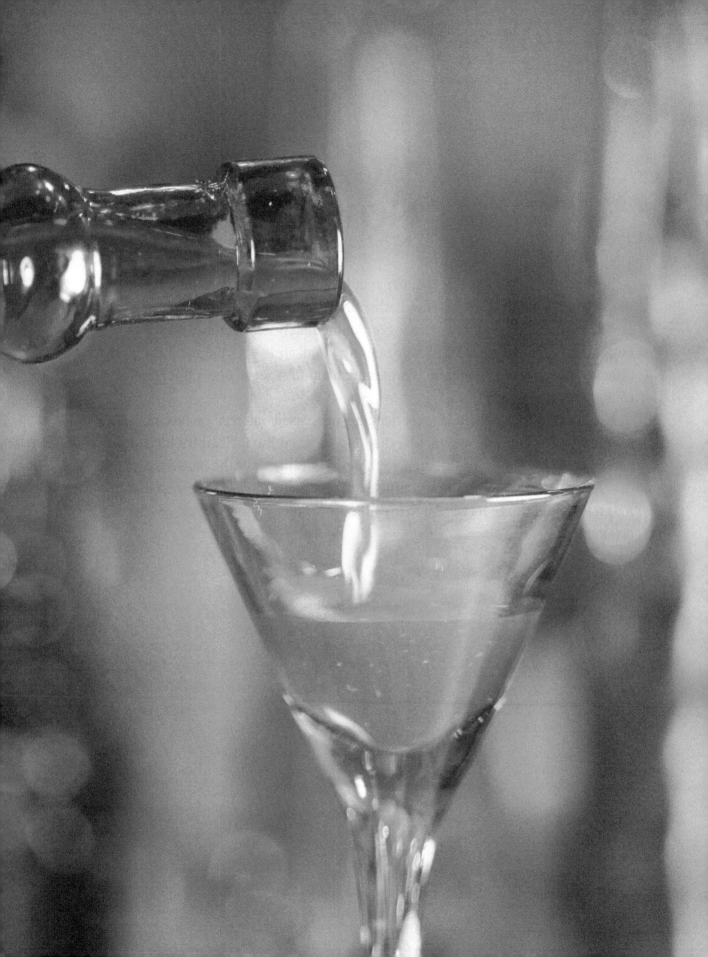

EUPHORIA ELIXIR

This magical libation has been tantalizing lovers for many moons. This is my previously guarded secret elixir recipe that increases sensation and intensifies orgasm.

---

4 oz damiana leaf
1 oz horny goat weed
2-3 whole dried vanilla beans
½ ounce rose petals

2 cinnamon sticks
7 ½ cups brandy
7 cups spring /filtered water
4 cups raw honey

Steep the damiana leaf, horny goat weed, rose, cinnamon and vanilla in brandy for 2 weeks, shaking the glass container every day with intention.

After at least 2 weeks filter the brandy out of the herbs. Store the infused brandy in a separate jar. Keep the strained brandy-soaked herbs in the same glass container and pour the water over top. Steep this water infusion for another 2 weeks, shaking daily.

After 2 weeks, filter/strain the water infusion off the plant material. Compost the herbs back to the Earth.

Take the water extraction and place it in a large saucepan. Bring it to a warm temperature, but be careful not to simmer or boil it! Once the liquid is warm, turn off the heat and add the honey. Stir until the honey dissolves completely.

Add the brandy infusion to the water/honey extract. Stir carefully for several minutes.

While stirring, this is the time to set your intention strongly into the cordial.

Store the cordial in bottles or glass jars for at least another 2 weeks before consuming. The longer it sits, the better it gets. I have some vintages that are over 15 years old, and they are getting better every day. That is if you can keep it around that long. This elixir tends to go fast. Euphoria elixir is always great with a lover, and it is a wonderful way to spice up social gatherings, too!

ALL NIGHT LONG!!! CHEWY CHOCOLATE POWER!

A super chocolaty chew to keep you going and going... in the bedroom or on the dance floor! Contains natural caffeine!

— ᎒ —

½ cup raw cacao powder
¼ cup raw mesquite powder
¼ cup raw Almond Butter, unsalted
¼ cup coconut sap syrup or raw agave nectar

1 tbs royal jelly in honey
2 tbs lacuma powder
½ tbs guarana powder
½ tbs kola nut powder
½ tsp vanilla extract
Pinch of sea salt

— ᎒ —

Mix the coconut sap syrup, almond Butter, royal jelly, vanilla extract and a pinch of sea salt together in a bowl. In a separate bowl combine the raw cacao powder, mesquite powder, lacuma, guarana and kola nut.

You can omit the kola nut, if you like, and double the amount of guarana instead. Mix the dry ingredients together by hand, breaking up clumps. Slowly add the wet ingredients into the dry, mixing with your hands.

The final "dough" should be sticky, but not too wet. You can add more lacuma powder if needed. Roll into balls or form into decorative shapes. Place in the refrigerator to harden. Serve chilled for the best flavor and texture.

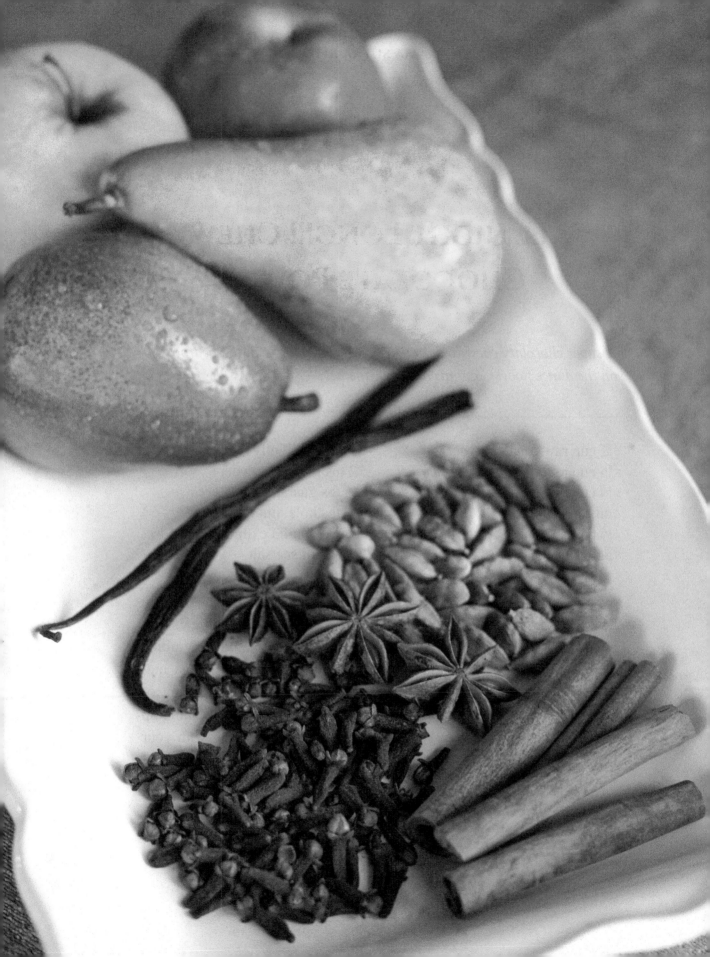

HARVEST LOVE BREW

This is a seasonal delight that I discovered one fall in the Berkshire Mountains in the USA, after a day of apple picking. It is a sweet and spicy drink that warms you from head to toe. Harvest Love Brew is wonderful to drink around a campfire or in front of a crackling fireplace!

---

6 cups apple juice, preferably freshly juiced or organic bottled
2 cups Pear juice, preferably freshly juiced or organic bottled
1/4 of a whole nutmeg seed
3 cinnamon sticks
6 cardamom pods, whole
5 whole cloves

1 star anise
¼ cup damiana leaf
2 strands of saffron
1 tsp dried rose petals
1 tbs catuaba bark

Freshly juice the apples and pears. If using bottled juices simply measure out and place into a pot on the stove. Add all the ingredients, except the saffron and the Rose, to the juice and simmer for 20 minutes, covered.

Remove from heat and add the saffron and the Rose and cover. Steep for another 5 minutes, strain and serve. Garnish with a cinnamon Stick in each cup!

—F3—

CHOCOLATE BLISS BALLS

My first and most popular recipe! I recommend eating at least 5 balls to really kick in the passion! This recipe can be successfully doubled if you want to make enough to share with a small crowd!

───────────────────── ❧ ─────────────────────

¼ cup raw cacao nibs, powdered
¼ cup raw cacao powder
1 tsp damiana leaf, powdered fine in small grinder or sifted with a strainer
1 tsp maca powder
½ tsp rhodiola powder
½ tsp ginseng powder
1 tsp guarana powder – optional
½ tsp lacuma fruit powder – optional

1 tsp cinnamon ½ tsp powdered rose
¼ tsp ginger
1/8 tsp cayenne – optional
Small pinch of salt
4 tbs of finely powdered cashews or pine nuts

1 tbs melted cacao butter
1 tbs melted coconut oil
¼ cup raw honey

───────────────────── ❧ ─────────────────────

Mix the herbs together with intention with your hands until all the colors are blended!

In a separate cup, blend the cacao butter, melted coconut oil and honey. From this blended mix of oil and sweetener, take 3 tbs and add it to the powdered herbs and chocolate. Store the rest of the liquid oil/sweetener in the refrigerator in an airtight container or lick off the body at another time.

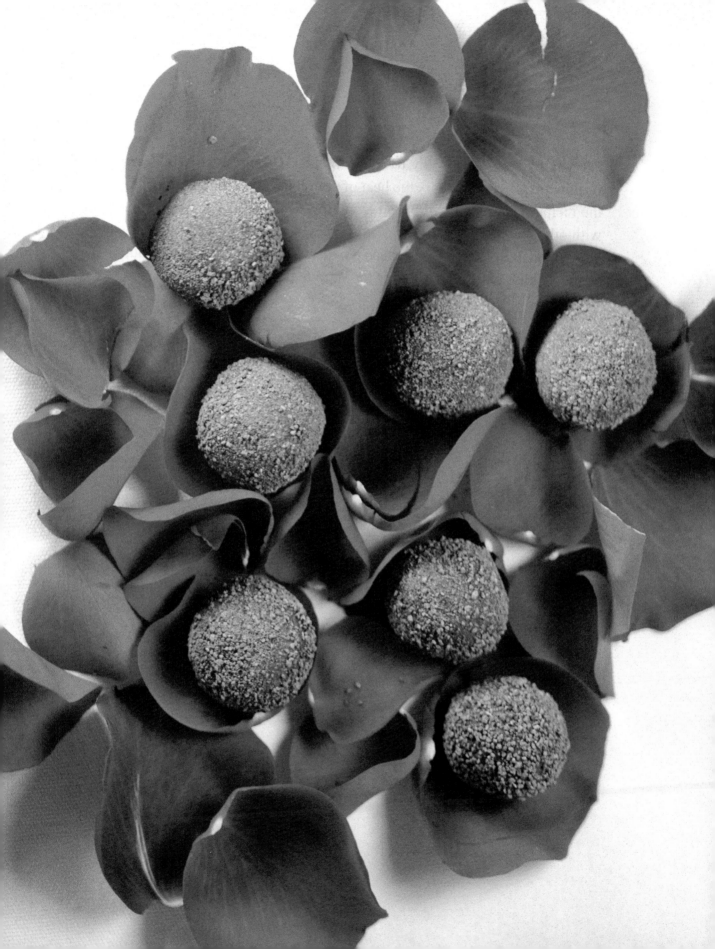

Mix by hand until ready to roll into balls. **Do not over mix! Very important!** If you over mix the heat of your hands will liquefy the oil in the recipe. The dough will become crumbly while your hands are slick with oil.

Optional: Roll the balls in cacao powder, cinnamon or dried coconut. Store the bliss balls in the freezer for up to 6 months!

Durian Mousse

If you love Durian, the exotic spiky fruit with an unusually pungent smell, you are going to flip over this amazing dessert. I recommend eating it off your lover's body if you're feeling adventurous.

1 cup fresh durian flesh
(remove stringy material if there
is any-you only want the soft,
custardy flesh)
¼ cup warm/hot water
1 tbs cacao powder

2 tbs cacao nibs/cacao beans,
powdered/ finely ground
1 tbs raw honey or coconut sap
syrup (optional)
1 tbs raw cacao butter, melted

Place the warm water into a blender. Add the cacao powder and cacao butter to the warm water and blend.

After blending add the powdered cacao nibs and honey if you choose to include it. Add the durian flesh in the blender or Cuisinart and pulse until smooth.

Chill in the fridge for an hour before serving. Durian Mousse is best when eaten off the body rather than a spoon.

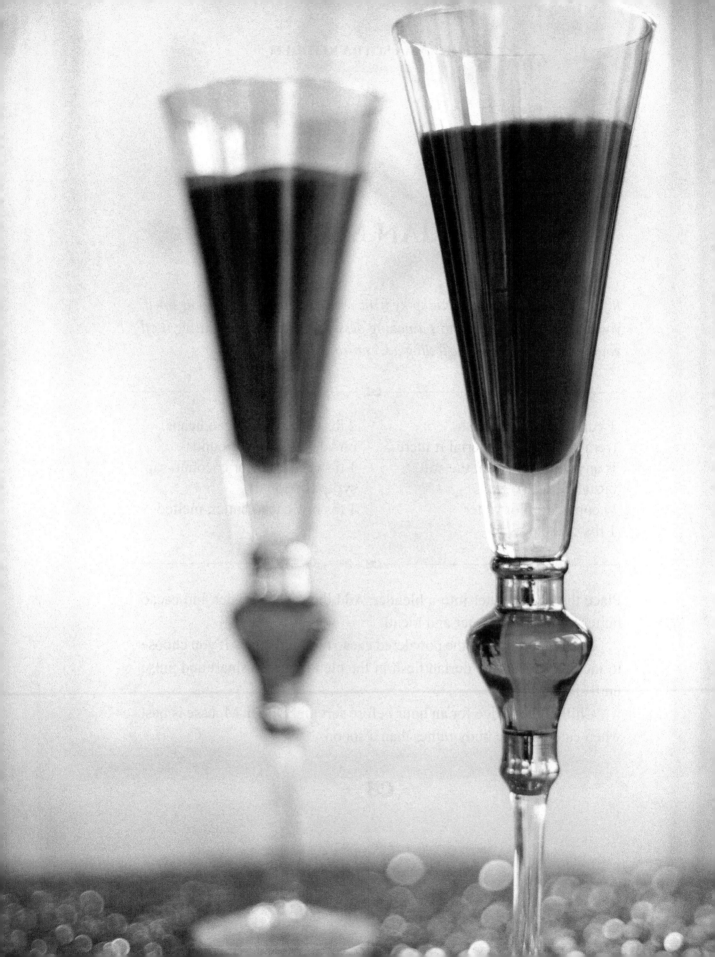

Choca Maca Coconut Quencher

A super tasty refreshing beverage that's great to keep close to the bed on a hot night!

Fresh coconut water from 2 young coconut s
3 tbs raw cacao powder
1 tsp coconut oil

1 tbs lacuma powder
1 tsp raw cacao nibs, powdered
3 tbs maca root powdered
1 tsp vanilla extract

Place all the ingredients in a blender and mix until well combined. Drink from a sexy glass or try sipping from a straw!

— ❧ —

DAMIANA LOVE TEA

This is my favorite libation for getting in the mood and enhancing orgasmic pleasure.

—— ❧ ——

3 cups water
½ cup damiana leaf
2 cinnamon sticks

2 tbs rose petals
½ cup horny goat weed leaf

—— ❧ ——

Bring the water to a boil with the cinnamon sticks. When the water is boiling, add damiana and the rose petals. Turn the heat off and cover with a lid. Steep 15 minutes. Strain and serve. Add honey or coconut sap for desired sweetness.

—— ❧ ——

LOVER'S CHAI

When making traditional chai the first thing to do is grind certain spices together to make a powdered masala chai spice mix. To do this we need the following spices in their whole form to grind them fresh to create our mix! To make the spice blend we need:

whole cinnamon sticks
whole green cardamom pods

black peppercorns
whole cloves

For the masala chai spice

½ tsp cinnamon, freshly powdered
½ tsp cardamom, freshly powdered

½ tsp clove, freshly powdered
1 tsp black pepper, freshly powdered

For the Lover's Chai

¼ tsp special masala chai spice mix
1 inch piece of fresh ginger, smashed
4 whole cloves
4 whole green cardamom pods, smashed open
3 strands of saffron
½ inch piece of dried vanilla Bean, sliced open or chopped up

3 tbs sugar/maple syrup/agave nectar/raw honey/coconut sap
2 cups almond milk, can substitute coconut, cow or goat milk
1 tbs black tea powder (contents of one tea bag, can substitute rooibos, tulsi or green tea)

Here is the recipe for the spice mix that I had to beg for in Rishikesh, India from everyone's favorite Chai stand in the market.

Freshly grind cinnamon sticks, whole cloves, whole green cardamom pods and whole black peppercorns, each one separately, in a coffee or spice grinder. Then add the amounts of each one listed back in the grinder and grind together until finely powdered. The final product is masala chai spice!

Now we are ready to make Lover's Chai!

Put the almond milk in a saucepan. Smash the fresh ginger and cardamom pods and with the whole cloves, saffron and vanilla, and put it all in a pot with the milk. Add the Tea powder or herbal replacement. Bring to a fast boil on the highest heat.

As soon as foam rises, lift the pot 1 foot off the flame and slowly bring back down onto the burner. Swirl the pot two times in a counterclockwise direction. Bring to a bubbling boil again. Wait until the foam rises, and repeat the lift and swirl technique.

For the third and last time, bring to a high rolling boil. This time wait for the foam to be a golden brown color. The smell should be strong now!

Lift and swirl, then put down and turn off the heat. Strain immediately into a pitcher and add sweetener. So yummy!

SEXY SMOKE

A smooth herbal smoking blend that relaxes the body and enhances sensitivity.

1tbs catnip dried leaf
1 tbs damiana dried leaf

Mix the catnip and damiana together and crush up. Roll a herbal cigarette with a rolling paper and smoke for a euphoric relaxing feeling without the nicotine.

Sexy Smoke can be a great way to relax after a stressful day, to set the mood, or to heighten the glow for those after sex smokers!

EROTIC CUISINE

Even without regarding active chemical constituents, foods can be considered an aphrodisiac by the way in which they are prepared, served and eaten. One of the most sensual food experiences I ever had was at a Moroccan restaurant where we sat on velvet pillows in a colorful silk tent. The food, spiced with aphrodisiac herbs, was excellent, but it was the sensuality of the environment and the presentation that sent us over the edge! All the food was eaten with our hands. We were in ecstasy by the time the meal was over after hours of feeding each other and licking fingers.

What makes a romantic dinner romantic? The answer is somewhat personal of course, but there are usually some common factors that create a foundation. Having the right atmosphere is very important. Candles, gentle lighting, perhaps a fire roaring in a fireplace and almost always, the right erotic music in the background sets the mood. The foods that are eaten play such an important role in building the passion and desire.

Perhaps somewhere out there someone finds burritos and cold corona with lime a truly romantic dinner, but at the risk of offense I am going to exclude that image from the majority's definition of the ideal romantic meal. While pizza and potato salad may romance our taste buds, they will do little to turn on our lovers from across the table. Finger foods, phallic shapes, juicy fruits, luscious sweets and easily reachable snacks are the essence of erotic cuisine. Refreshing beverages that tingle the taste buds and send yummy sensations down the throat are essential! Try a few of these…

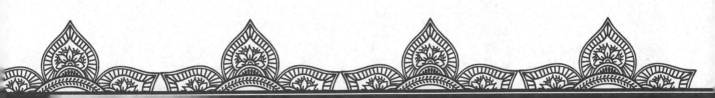

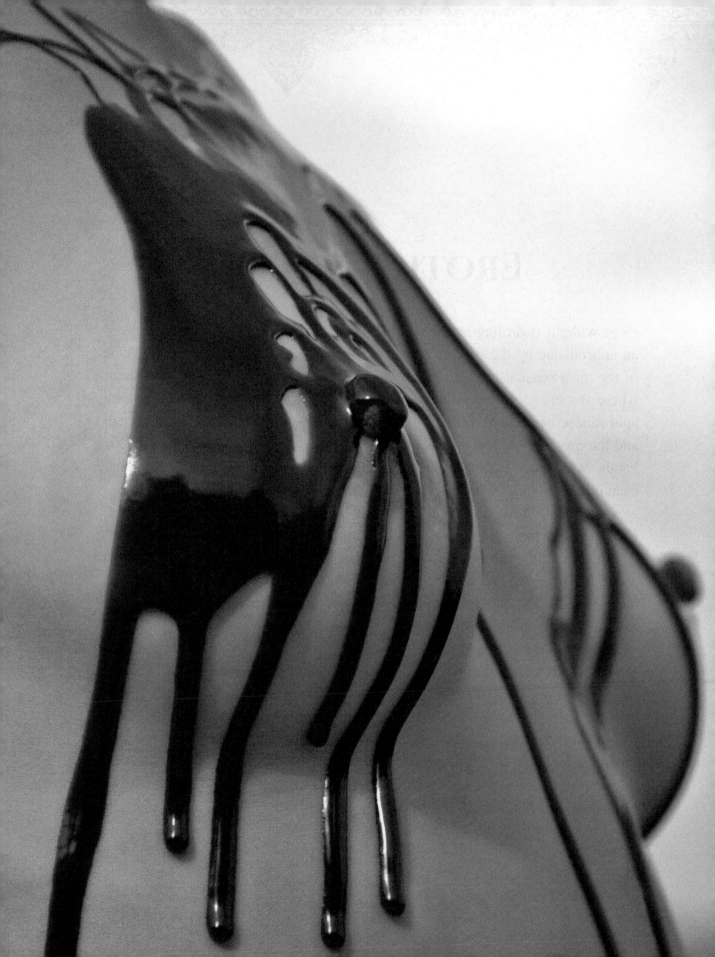

CHOCOLATE NIPPLE PASTE

1 tbs raw cacao nibs, ground/powdered in a Vitamix or coffee grinder
8 tbs raw cacao powder
1 tbs raw cacao butter, liquid
1 tbs raw coconut oil, liquid
Dash of sea salt
Optional:
1/8 tsp cinnamon powder

½ cup raw honey or coconut sap syrup
1 tbs royal jelly in honey
½ tsp vanilla extract
2 tbs goji berries, ground up into a rough powder

Dash of chili powder – careful now! Remember this may be on someone's nipples!

In a mixing bowl combine the powdered cacao nibs, cacao powder, sea salt and any optional spices. In a separate bowl mix the cacao butter, coconut oil, coconut sap syrup, royal jelly and vanilla extract until well blended. Slowly add the liquid into the dry ingredients stirring as you pour. When you grind the goji berries add a ½ tsp of cacao powder to keep them from sticking. Add the goji berries last, mix well and store in a decorative glass jar for bedside application.

CHOCOLATE ALMOND YUM BARS

Super yummy nutritious chocolate covered delights! I keep them in my freezer and reach for one when I'm craving sweets. They are great for sustaining energy and providing essential nutrients. Did I mention they're delicious?!!

———————— ✄ ————————

2 cups almonds, ideally soaked and dried – or just raw
¼ cup ground flaxseed
½ cup dates plus one date
1/3 cup dried coconut ground up
½ cup pumpkin seed butter, or raw almond butter or raw tahini
½ tsp unrefined sea salt
½ cup coconut oil, soft not liquid

2-3 tsp vanilla extract
1 tsp mesquite pod powder
1 tsp cinnamon powder
1 tbs maca powder
5 ounces cacao paste
½ tsp vanilla extract
2 tbs (1.5 ounces) raw honey

———————— ✄ ————————

Grind the flax seeds up into a coarse powder using a magic bullet blender, Vitamix, Cuisinart or hand grinder. Place the almonds, the coconut flakes and the ground flax seeds in Vitamix or Cuisinart and blend. I like the texture medium/fine ground but if you are a chunky kinda lover you can adjust as you prefer. Pour into a bowl and add 1 tbs chia seeds. Add mesquite, salt, cinnamon and maca. Put the dates, nut butter, coconut oil, not melted but soft, and vanilla extract in the Vitamix and blend.

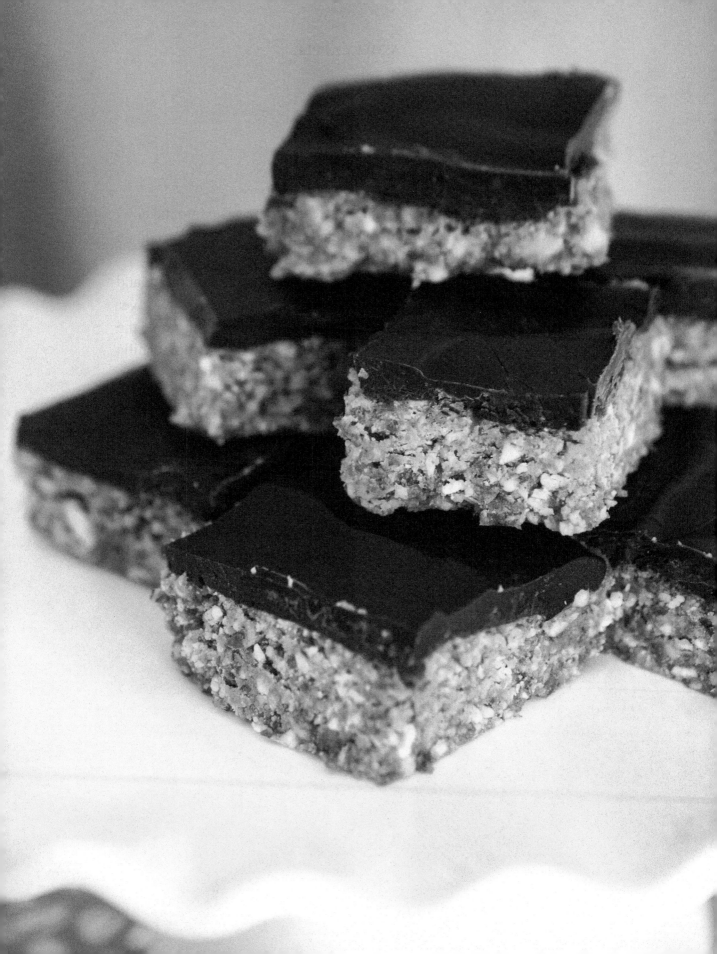

This should make a thick creamy paste. Pour the paste into the bowl with the powdered nuts and mix by hand. Press into wax paper lined square pan, 8"x8". Place in the freezer while making chocolate.

For the chocolate coating, weigh 5 ounces of raw cacao paste and melt in a double boiler on medium heat. You can place a glass bowl over a pot of simmering water if you don't have a double boiler. Once the paste is melted, remove from heat and let cool slightly. Add the vanilla extract and honey, stirring continuously. Don't add the honey too soon to the cacao paste after you remove from the heat or it will harden funny and curdle. Wait for the chocolate to be warm, thick and still fluid.

Remove the nut base from the freezer and using a spatula or knife spread the chocolate over the bars evenly. Place in the freezer for 10 minutes ONLY. Long enough for the chocolate to cool but not completely harden.

Using a sharp long knife, lifting the bars out of the pan by the wax paper, slice into squares. Place in a Tupperware and store in the fridge or freezer.

LICKABLE LINGAM TINGLE POTION

This is yummy edible massage oil intended for the male genitals that heats up the skin when you blow on it with hot breath. The peppermint and kava create a unique tingly sensation.

1 tbs vegetable glycerin
1 tbs raw coconut oil
½ tsp vanilla extract

1 tsp Kava Kava tincture
1 drop (only one!!!) peppermint essential oil

In a small mixing bowl combine all the ingredients and mix thoroughly with sensual strokes. Be careful when applying this to the male genitalia…too much tingle can be a turn off!

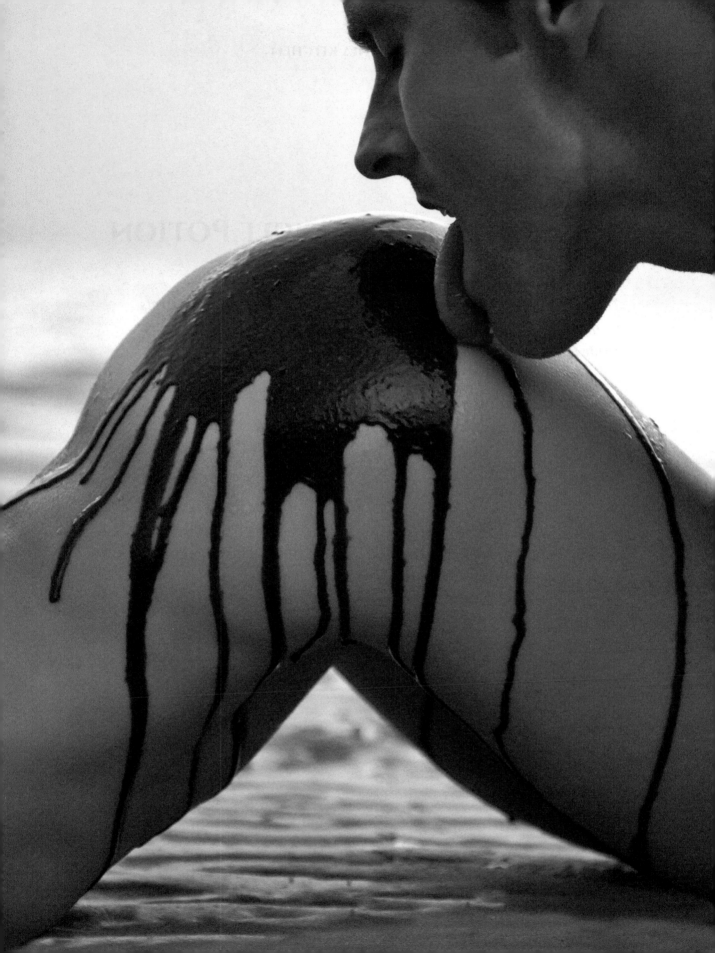

CHOCOLATE BODY SYRUP

¼ cup raw cacao butter, melted
¼ cup raw honey or coconut sap syrup

3 tbs raw cacao powder
½ tsp vanilla extract

Blend the melted cacao butter and the sweetener together. Mix in the vanilla. Stir in the cacao powder and get ready to lick!

MAGIC MANGO WANDS

These lead to all kinds of fun! Get creative and place them anywhere on the body you want to taste mango sweetness.

---

1 fresh mango
vanilla extract

Cut the mango into long strips (thick french fry cut) then place in a flat dish with sides and pour the vanilla over the mango. Marinate in the refrigerator for an hour.

Place mango by the lovemaking area to be used on the genitals of the woman. Cool mango slices are stimulating on the yoni, vagina. Half the fun is eating the mango slices off the body! Mmm… mango flavored yoni!

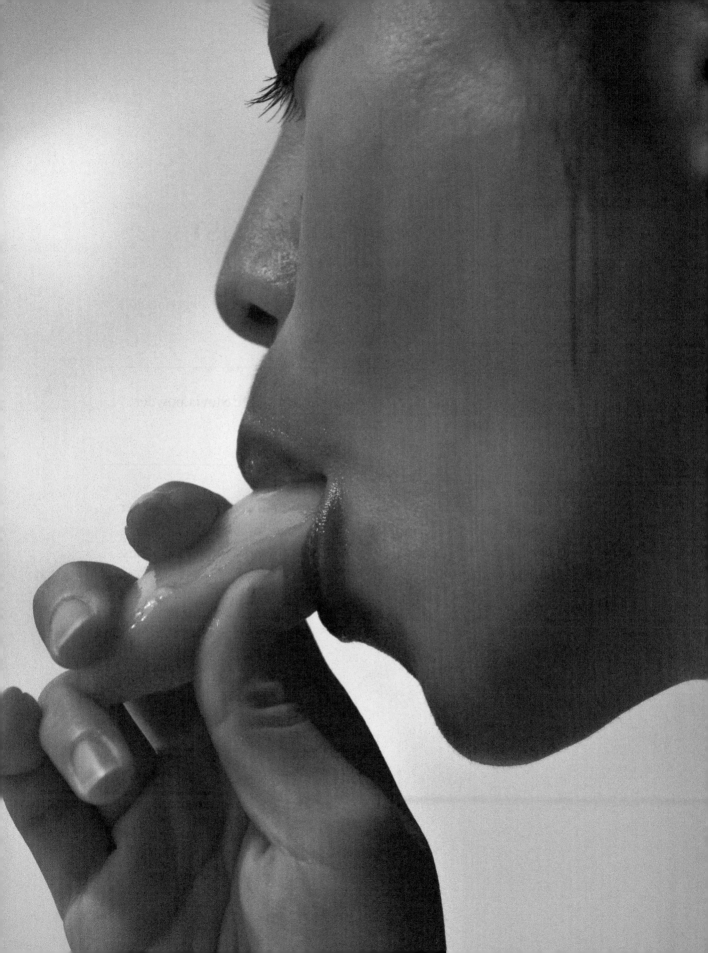

YUM YUM YONI DUST

Leave a sensual hint of rose dusted on your thighs, a sweet lingering note of what's to come…

1 tbs Arrowroot powder
½ tsp powdered roses

1/16 tsp White Stevia powder

Mix all the ingredients together and store in a small decorative container. Apply to the inner thighs and yoni with a feather for a luxurious feeling. Yoni dust leaves a delicate trace of rose aroma and a subtle sweetness when licked!

—❧—

CLOUD 9 BODY BUTTER

It is hard to keep this stuff around due to the extreme sensation of ecstasy it causes in the mouth…

½ cup raw coconut butter
1 tbs raw cacao nibs
4 tbs raw cacao powder

3 tbs raw honey or coconut sap syrup
1 tsp vanilla extract

(Coconut butter is a very unique ingredient, not to be confused with raw coconut oil. coconut butter is a blend of the oil and the meat of the coconut and tastes slightly sweet and smooth. It is sold in most organic health food stores in the USA.)

Warm the coconut butter in a double boiler to a paste consistency. Do not overheat! Add the honey or coconut sap syrup and blend well. Mix in the vanilla extract. Add the raw cacao powder and mix well. Finally, add the raw cacao nibs and mix.

Store in a glass jar or eat right out of the bowl. Smear on body, desserts and fingers, or eat right off the spoon! I like to mold Cloud 9 Body butter in the shape of a heart using a cookie cutter. I fill the mold and place it in the refrigerator to harden up some before removing. It is hard to keep this stuff around due to the extreme sensation of ecstasy it causes in the mouth…

BLISS STUFFED DATES

These sweet, sexy treats are purrfect for the bedside table.

---

8 medjool dates
1 cup pine nuts
½ whole vanilla bean or ½ tsp vanilla extract
¼ cup warm water
1 tsp royal jelly

2 tbs raw honey or coconut sap syrup
1 tbs raw cacao powder – optional
raw cacao nibs
Pinch of sea salt

Soak the vanilla bean pod in ¼ cup warm water for 30 minutes to soften it. De-seed the dates by splitting down one side, removing the seed and separating it into two halves. Set the dates aside.

Blend the pine nuts, raw honey, royal jelly, optional raw cacao powder, soaked vanilla bean and the water it was soaked in, and a pinch of sea salt together in blender/Vitamix/Cuisinart until creamy. Fill each date half with the pine nut paste and arrange on a plate.

Optional: sprinkle with cacao nibs. Place the plate within reach of your sacred sex space.

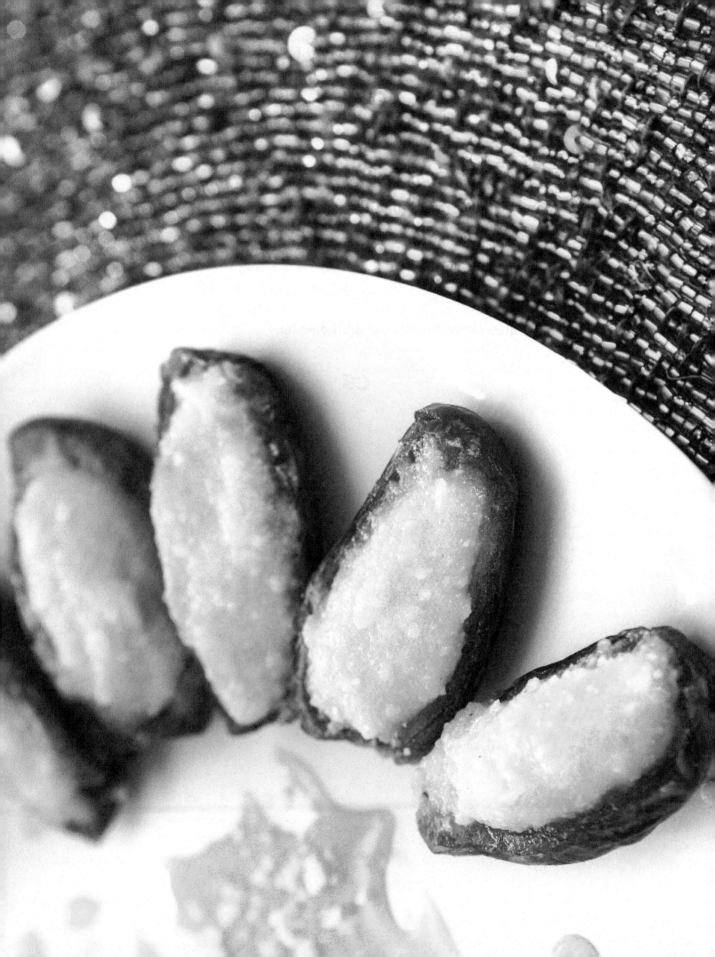

Quick and Dirty version for filling:

1 cup Cashew nut butter	1 tsp royal jelly
½ tsp vanilla extract	Pinch of salt
2 tbs raw honey	

Mix all the ingredients together and fill date halves.

APPLE PIE SQUARES

A wonderful dessert or bedside snack to help sweeten the mood.

For the crust
1 cup medjool dates, pitted
¼ cup Black Mission figs, dried, chopped and de-stemmed
¼ cup almonds, chopped in small chunks
¼ cup Cashews, ground finely into a powder
¼ cup Sesame seeds, ground roughly
1-2 tbs dry shredded coconut, depending on your coconut adoration
Pinch of sea salt

For the pie filling
3 cups Granny Smith apples, chopped in small chunks
1 tbs fresh lemon juice
½ cup cashews powdered
1 tsp cinnamon powder
8 dates, pitted
½ cup warm water

Decoration/ Garnish:
almonds
goji berries
apple slices
dried fig slices

Place the dates and Figs into a Cuisinart or Blender and blend until it resembles one big ball of sweet goo. Sprinkle in the almonds and mix. Add the Cashew powder and Sesame seeds. Mix well and then add the coconut. Mix again until everything is blended.

You can choose to mix the crust by hand, to add more sensuality and loving energy. Press the mixture into a pie plate or into a square pan. Refrigerate while preparing the filling.

Soak the dates in the warm water and put aside. Place the apple chunks in a bowl and sprinkle the lemon juice over them. Toss lightly. Mix the cashew powder and cinnamon together in a separate bowl. Sprinkle over the apples and toss.

Blend the soaked dates and the water used for soaking them in a blender.

Finally, add the thick date paste to the apples and mix well. Pour the filling into the crust and smooth the top.

Decorate with a garnish and place in the refrigerator.

The apple pie tastes best if served within a couple hours. It will taste great the next day, but the apples will have lost some of their crispness.

OH MY LICKABLE GOD!

Wow. Seriously divine deliciousness! Lick this off body parts and watch out!!

1 tbs raw cacao butter, melted
1 tbs raw coconut oil, melted

4 tbs raw honey
½ tsp vanilla extract

Blend ingredients together until smooth.

Oh My Lickable God is one of the most delicious edible body syrups you will ever try! It melts in your mouth while opening up your body to more sensuous experiences.

CHOCOLATE HEARTS

This is the recipe I serve with my elixirs, partnering luscious libations with dark chocolate deliciousness. I have kept it a secret until now. To make purr-fect raw chocolate every time it is important to weigh the ingredients. Most kitchen supply stores will carry inexpensive scales that weigh in ounces.

ᘓ

8 ounces raw cacao butter
6.5 ounces raw cacao powder, sifted
½ cup coconut sap syrup
½ tsp white stevia powder, optional
1 tsp vanilla extract
pinch of salt

Optional:
2 tbs almonds, roughly chopped
        or
1 drop peppermint essential oil
        or
1 tbs goji berries, roughly chopped
coarse ground sea salt

ᘓ

If you are adding optional ingredients to flavor the chocolates place them inside each heart mold and set aside so they are ready when you pour the chocolate over. There will be a short window to work with the liquid chocolate and you want to have everything ready.

Melt the cacao butter gently in a metal or glass bowl sitting on top a pot of boiling water, like a double boiler. Turn off the heat.

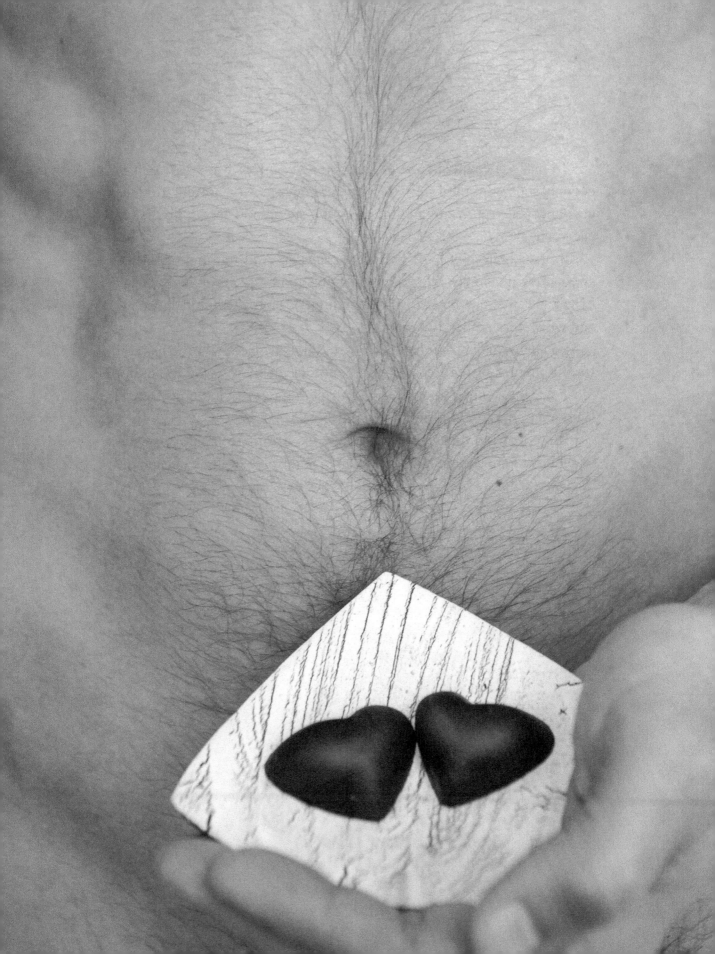

To make coconut sap syrup, add 2 tbs of boiling water to 1 cup of coconut sugar. Stir until smooth. Some granules may be present. Add the coconut sap syrup, vanilla extract and the stevia powder to the melted cacao butter. Whisk for 30 seconds.

In a separate bowl sift the cacao powder. Add the melted cacao/sweetener mix slowly, whisking while you combine. Sprinkle the pinch of salt and any other flavorings (peppermint oil) into the liquid chocolate and whisk for another 30 seconds.

Pour into small plastic heart shaped molds and place in the refrigerator for 30 minutes or until hardened. Do not let them sit in the molds for too long, the condensation from the fridge may alter the consistency. Remove from the fridge and pop the chocolates out.

I like to wrap them in decorative colored foils to create suspense when unwrapping them later! Store them in airtight zip lock bags in the refrigerator for up to a week, or the freezer for a month.

ROSE LEMONADE

½ cup freshly squeezed lemon juice
3 cups water
4 tbs maple syrup or raw honey

1 drop!!!! rose essential oil (rose otto – steam distilled)
garnish: rose petals

Mix lemon juice and water, stirring with intention!

Add one drop – and only one drop – of rose essential oil to the honey or maple syrup in a separate cup and stir. Add the rose infused sweetener to the lemon juice.

Chill in refrigerator until ready to serve. Garnish with rose petals.

—CB—

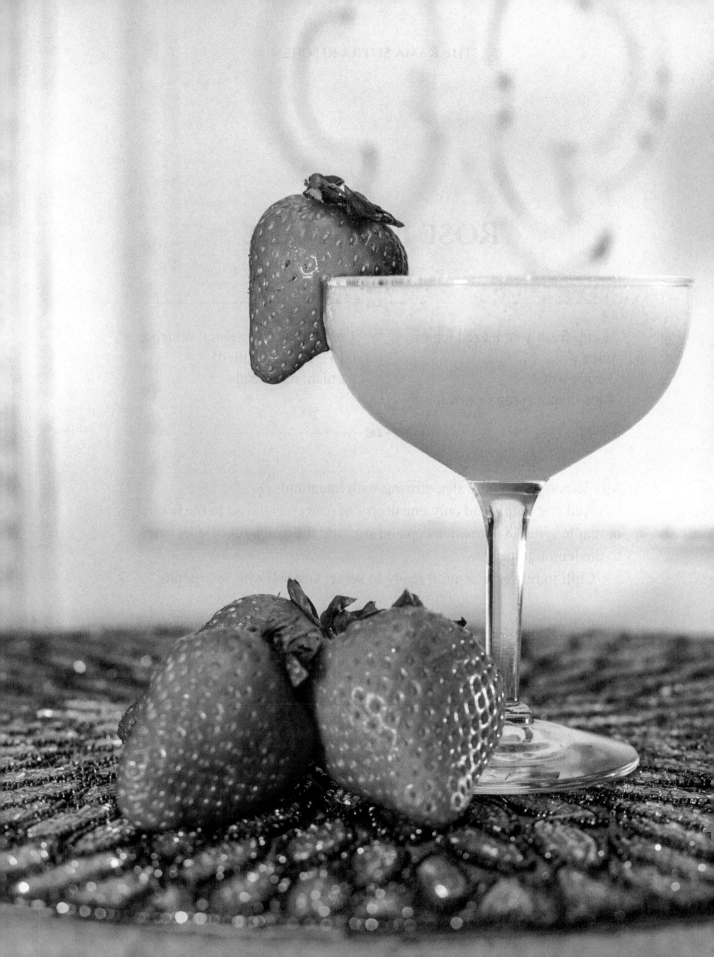

STRAWBERRY ALMOND DELIGHT

2 cups of fresh raw almond milk
(see recipe on page 106")
1 cup fresh strawberries

3 dates or 2 tbs raw honey
½ tsp vanilla extract
or ½ vanilla bean

Place all the ingredients in a blender and pulse until fully pureed.

Sip sensually on a hot steamy afternoon or in between lovemaking sessions for a quick blood sugar boost with sustaining energy!

RAW ALMOND MILK

---

1 cup almonds soaked in 4 cups
filtered/spring water for 6-12
hours

3 cups water
pinch of sea salt
½ tsp vanilla extract

Drain off soak water and place almonds, sea salt and vanilla in a blender
with 3 cups water. Blend until creamy. Strain through a nut milk bag,
fine mesh strainer, or cheesecloth.

Almond milk will keep for three days in the refrigerator.

—&—

CHOCOLATE MINT MOUSSE

A refreshing, rich chocolate mousse full of healthy fats, minerals and sensual flavors begging to be eaten off the body!

1 cup fresh coconut water
1 ½ – 2 cups young coconut Meat
¼ cup raw cacao nibs, finely ground
½ cup cacao powder
1 tbs raw cacao butter, melted

1/3 tsp vanilla extract
¼ cup raw honey or coconut sap syrup
2 drops peppermint essential oil, food grade or ½ tsp peppermint extract

Place all the ingredients in the blender and pulse until completely smooth.

Pour into a sealable container and place in the freezer. Wait until the Mousse has set, 3-5 hours ONLY. Remove and devour or place in the fridge for later consumption.

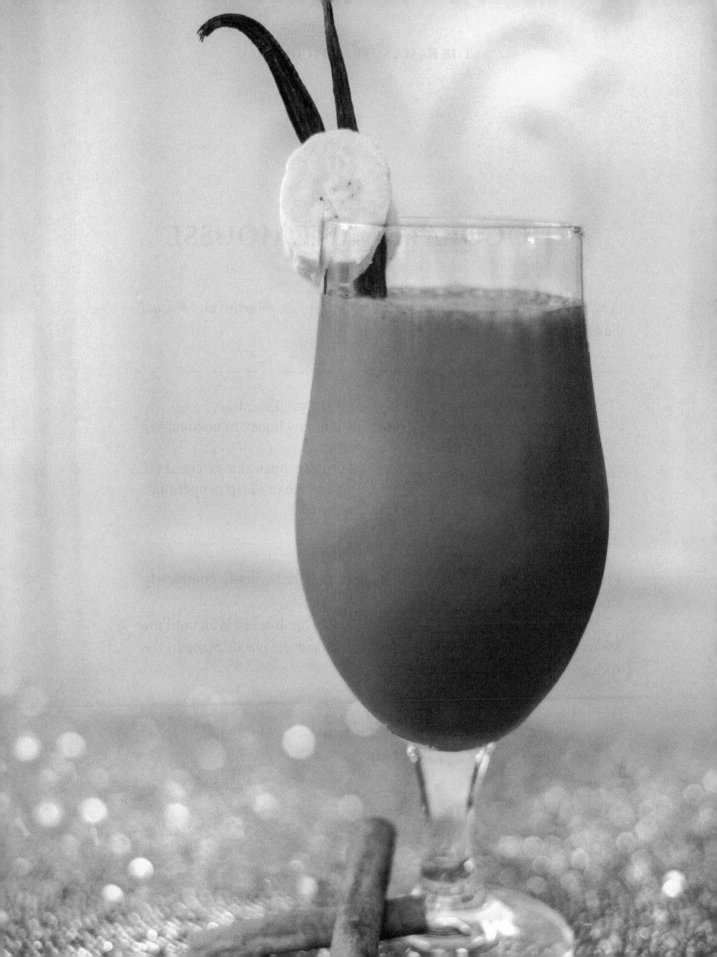

KAMA SUTRA SHAKE

4 tbs raw Chocolate powder
3 tbs coconut sap syrup or raw honey
1 tsp royal jelly
2 cups raw almond milk

3 Frozen Bananas
½ vanilla bean or ½ tsp vanilla extract
½ tsp cinnamon
1 tbs maca powder

Frozen bananas are easy to prepare: Simply peel the bananas and place them in a zip lock bag for several hours or overnight. Make sure to squeeze the air out of the bag before sealing to prevent freezer snow on the fruit.

To make the shake, put all the ingredients in the blender and pulse till smooth.

This is my favorite drink to serve at a social gathering! Be prepared, everyone usually wants seconds!

LIPS OF THE GODDESS

In the novel, Siddhartha, Kamala, the radiant courtesan who inspired every man with passion and desire, had her lips compared to two halves of a freshly cut fig. The ripe cut fruit is erotic and exotic on a decorated plate, perfect for seducing or snacking!

---

6 fresh figs   ½ cup raw honey
vanilla syrup   2 whole vanilla beans

Slice the vanilla beans down the middle and spread the seed open. Cut into small pieces and place with the sweetener in a blender. Blend until smooth.

Cut the figs in half and place on a plate with fresh mint or hyssop leaves. Drizzle some of the vanilla syrup over the figs and some on the plate.

Eat with your fingers! Licking and sucking the sticky sweetness from your lover's hands is encouraged!

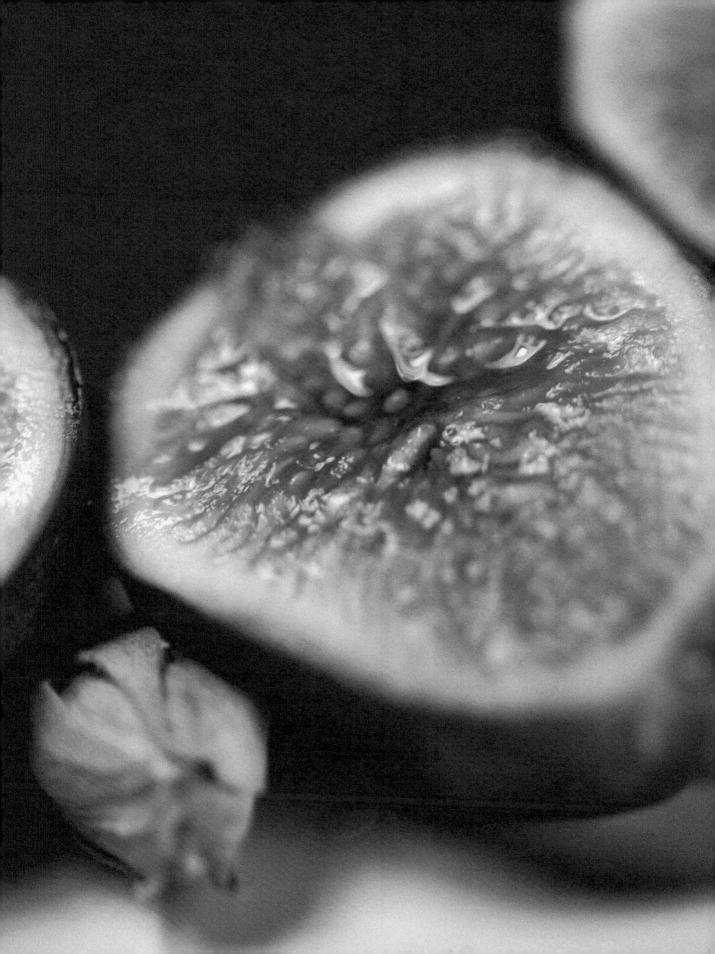

Seduction and the Art of Temptation

The greatest aphrodisiac of all is the mind. The easiest and simplest practice is that of temptation. If we can successfully build desire and passion by tempting and teasing then we have already ignited the most powerful aphrodisiac effects. Besides decorating our lovemaking space and arranging a ready supply of treats and refreshments, we can prepare by planning the slowest, most excruciatingly tempting way to offer them.

The most important rule in seduction and in passion is to take our time. The slower and more deliberately we move and the longer we draw it out, the more desire grows and energy builds. Building sexual energy is the most important way to experience extreme sensual bliss and pleasure. The more sexual energy we build, the more likely we are to hear afterwards our lover just had the best sex of his/her life. They will sigh blissfully and thank God that we are in his/her life. The Kama Sutra instructs the man to wait for certain signs, such as moaning and sighing, restless body movements and toe curling before actually penetrating the woman. I offer the same sort of advice to both men and women when it comes to aphrodisiacs. Use the aphrodisiacs and sensual foods to create a teasing mood. Feed them to one another slowly. Offer a treat with your hands and pull away before they can have any. The more wanting you build, the more passion, and the greater the pleasure. Who wants to try?

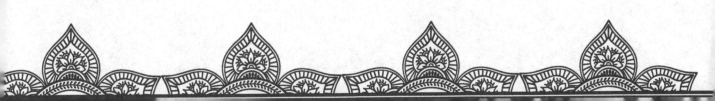

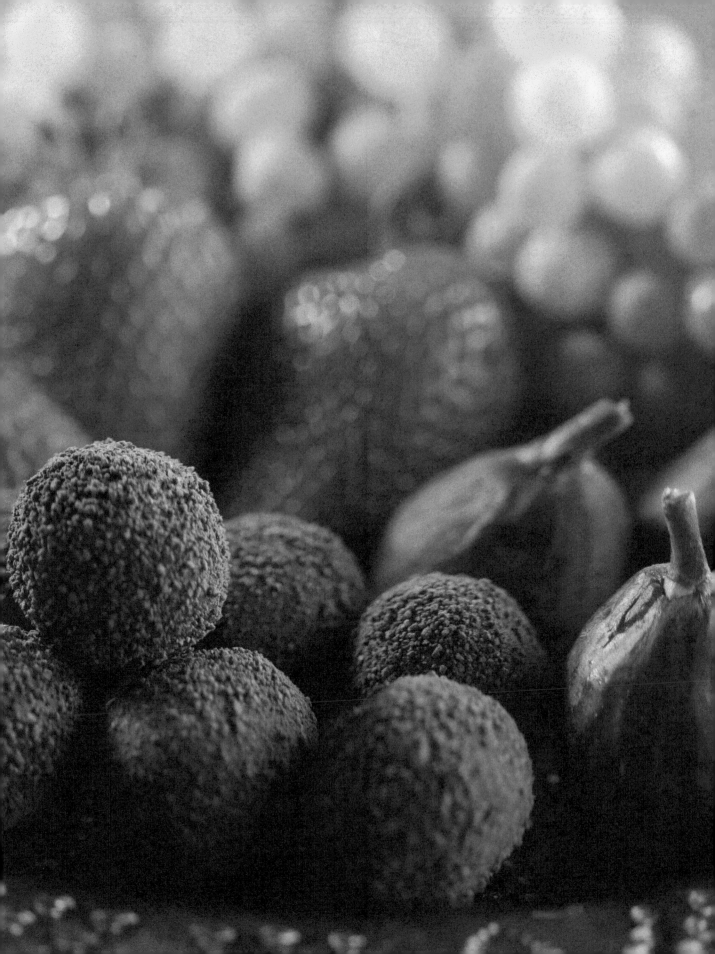

Sexy Suggestions for Seduction

- Blindfold your lover and wave various delicacies under his/her nose. You may want to try rose petals, chocolate, coffee beans, vanilla, your perfume or cologne, lavender, orange slices, ylang ylang essential oil, etc. Try rubbing a little honey, chocolate and orange juice on their lips for them to lick. Surprise your lover at the end with your own lips.
- Take some cold mango slices from the fridge and run one over your lover's body. Lick along the trail of mango juice. This technique is especially wonderful on women. The feeling of a cold mango slice gently running over and in-between the lips of the yoni is amazing!!! The partner gets to enjoy the body juicy with mango flavor and yumminess!
- Lay your lover down and very slowly run a feather over their entire body for 10 minutes. Tease the underarms, behind the knees and in between the thighs for brief encounters to create shivers and chills!

Here is a sample plan for preparing your space for an amazing evening!

Decoration:
- Sprinkle rose petals on the floor and bed
- Use aromatherapy oil in a diffuser (rose, ylang ylang, cinnamon, vanilla, patchouli)
- Burn incense
- Place feathers by the bed (peacock feathers are very soft and beautiful)
- Arrange candles at different heights throughout the room-by the bed, along the floor
- Drape sensuous fabrics or scarves over lamps and hang them from the ceiling. You can create a Bedouin style tent around the bed to add another flare of romance.

- Buy some new sheets that feel soft and luxurious, made from materials like satin, silk, very fine cotton or my new eco favorite, 100% bamboo.
- Choose sensual background music to play continually
- Place fresh flowers in several vases around the room. (Make sure your lover isn't allergic to them!)
- Put drinks and sweet treats on both sides of the bed and in other places around the room. Something should be in reach wherever you go!

Drinks:
- Pitcher of water and two cups that are specially designed. Perhaps they are delicate or artistic. Whatever you feel best inspires the mood.
- A carafe of hot herbal aphrodisiac tea like Damiana Love Tea
- Freshly squeezed juice or the water from Thai young coconuts can be very refreshing. I like fresh orange or apple juice the best. Apples are known for being especially good at stimulating the sexual energy center.
- Chocolate Maca Almond Milk or Strawberry Almond Delight

Sweet Treats:
- Stuffed dates
- Magic Mango Wands
- sliced fruit
- Chocolate Bliss Balls
- Chocolate Durian Mousse
- Edible body syrups and butters
- Chocolate Nipple Paste – always good to keep a jar by the bed!

CONCLUSION

In Tantra yoga the body is considered a divine temple for the soul to reside in. The act of making love is the merging of the two energies of the universe, Shiva and Shakti, Yin and Yang, Masculine and Feminine. It is in this union of energy that we find ecstatic states of bliss.

Making love together with our lover can be an opportunity to open our hearts and experience the deepest aspects of love and truth. If we come to "bed" with such an intention, it is easy to cultivate. When we see the divinity and beauty of our lover, sex becomes sacred.

The aphrodisiac plants and foods that help create that sacred sexual energy are indeed gifts from nature. In my experience, aphrodisiacs can help us open to our sensual nature and inspire worship in our lovemaking.

The most important thing is to have fun and enjoy experimenting! May you love more, feel more and dance divinely under the sheets of passion and pleasure!

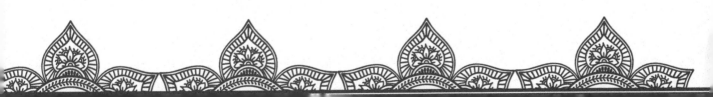

INDEX OF RECIPES

You can read more about Ashley's

courses on her website and hear about

upcoming books and appearances.

www.ashleyapple.com

CPSIA information can be obtained
at www.ICGtesting.com
Printed in the USA
LVOW06s2039150217
524360LV00008B/308/P

9 780615 998930